A NOTE ON THE EDITOR

Mona Eltahawy (she/her) is a feminist author, commentator and disruptor of patriarchy. Her first book, *Headscarves and Hymens: Why the Middle East Needs a Sexual Revolution* (2015), targeted patriarchy in the Middle East and North Africa, and her second, *The Seven Necessary Sins for Women and Girls* (2019), took her disruption worldwide. Her commentary has appeared in media around the world, and she is editor-in-chief and essayist for the newsletter FEMINIST GIANT.

ALSO BY MONA ELTAHAWY

*Headscarves and Hymens:
Why the Middle East Needs a Sexual Revolution*

The Seven Necessary Sins for Women and Girls

BLOODY HELL!

ADVENTURES IN MENOPAUSE
FROM AROUND THE WORLD

EDITED BY MONA ELTAHAWY

unbound

First published in 2025

Unbound
c/o TC Group, 6th Floor King's House, 9–10 Haymarket,
London SW1Y 4BP
www.unbound.com
All rights reserved

© Mona Eltahawy, 2025
Individual work © respective contributors, 2025
Illustrations © Sheyam Ghieth, 2025

The right of Mona Eltahawy to be identified as the editor of this work has been asserted in accordance with Section 77 of the Copyright, Designs and Patents Act, 1988. No part of this publication may be copied, reproduced, stored in a retrieval system, or transmitted, in any form or by any means without the prior permission of the publisher, nor be otherwise circulated in any form of binding or cover other than that in which it is published and without a similar condition being imposed on the subsequent purchaser.

While every effort has been made to trace the owners of copyright material reproduced herein, the publisher would like to apologise for any omissions and will be pleased to incorporate missing acknowledgements in any further editions.

Typeset in 10/14pt Sabon LT Pro by Jouve (UK), Milton Keynes

A CIP record for this book is available from the British Library

ISBN 978-1-80018-371-1 (paperback)
ISBN 978-1-80018-372-8 (ebook)

Printed and bound in Great Britain by Bell & Bain Ltd, Glasgow

1 3 5 7 9 8 6 4 2

With love and solidarity for your transition

With special thanks to the patrons of this book:
Ruth Ann Harnisch
Ruth Ann Subach

Contents

Introduction by Mona Eltahawy   xiii

The Menopause: When We Are Free
Marilyn Muthoni Kamuru   1

The Yellies
Simi Hoque   16

Bits of Flesh: For Anarcha – From Enslavement
to Menopause
Omisade Burney-Scott   28

Gender, What Even Was That? Or, Diary of a Chest
Tania Glyde   41

The Curse of Puberty
Jenn Salib Huber   54

Don't Bring a Flashlight to the Brain Fog
Sonora Jha   67

Lost Pages from the Lore of Menses /
كتابات الفائضات في نزهات الحائضات
Mohja Kahf   79

My Bleeding Life
Emmett Jack Lundberg   93

I Don't Like Being Late: An Experience of
Perimenopause From Turkey
Aslı Alpar (translated by Canan Marasligil)   105

This Is Going Somewhere Good
Ann Marie McQueen   121

The Body Changes: Menopause Brings Change
Kimberly Dark   134

Sex and the Menopausal Vagina in the Suburbs
Susan Cole   148

Where Do I End? Wherever I Begin
Una Mullally   162

My Mother, the Menopause and Me
Nana Darkoa Sekyiamah   174

Feeling OldCute. Might Delete Later
Abeer Y. Hoque   183

A Field Guide to Menopause
M'kali-Hashiki   199

Free Fall
Syd Yang   213

Afterword   227
Notes   237
Acknowledgements   243
Supporters   245
A Note on the Type   254

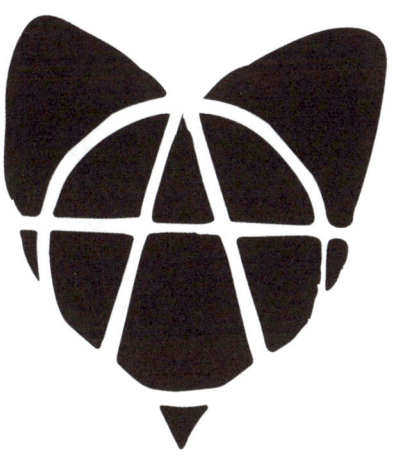

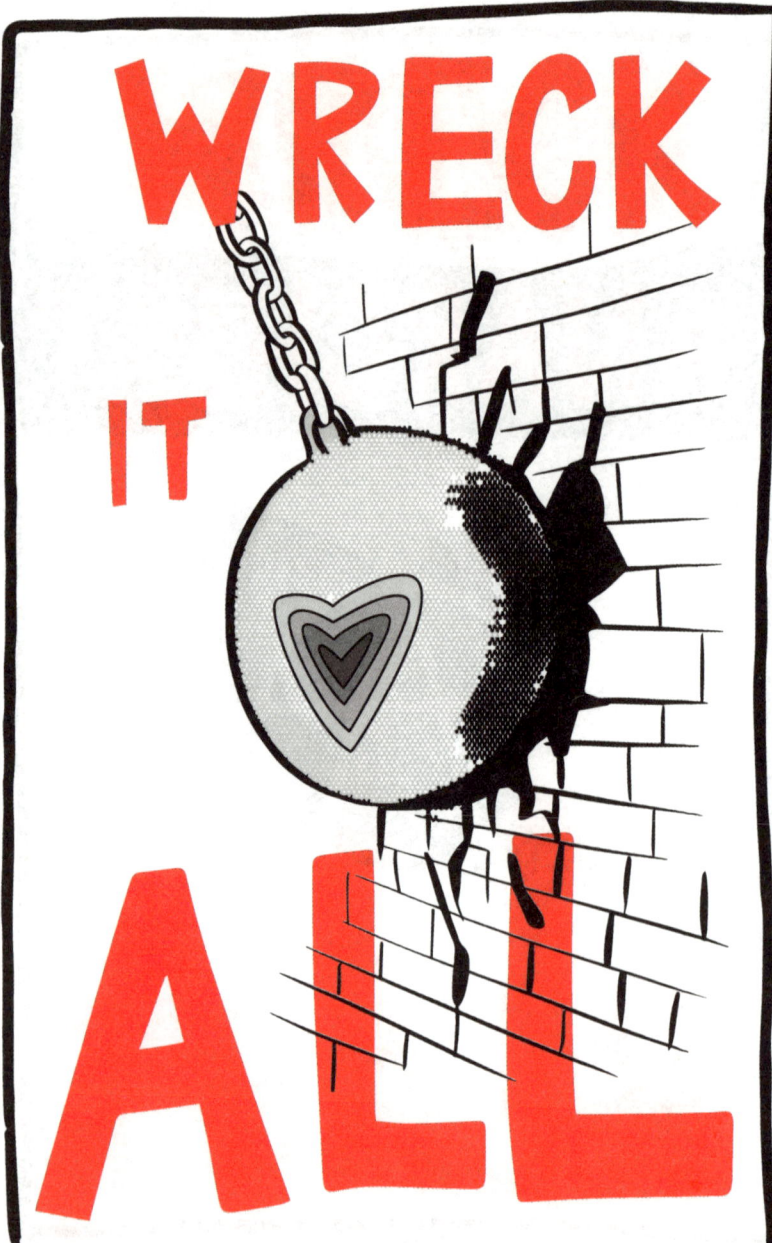

Introduction

Mona Eltahawy

I found out almost by chance that perimenopause – the time leading up to menopause – can last up to fourteen years. At first I thought, 'Are you fucking kidding me?' And that quickly turned to, 'How the hell did I not know that?'

How was a feminist like me so ignorant about menopause? Was I not paying attention?

There wasn't much to pay attention to when those first flickers of perimenopause started teasing/testing/taunting my knowledge. When one by one those impacts of the menopause transition began kicking me around as if they were running a relay over my body, it was to social media that I turned. I often just had to say, 'My fucking perimenopause,' on the platform formerly known as Twitter for dozens upon dozens of people to respond with their, 'Oh my God! I feel understood!' And it was there on social media that kind strangers, as well as friends who'd been paying a bit more attention than I had been, recommended accounts to follow. That led to a deep dive into the menopause transition and also new friendships and camaraderie with the founders of those dedicated menopause accounts. Several of them were kind enough to accept my invitation to contribute to this anthology. I have learned a lot from them and I am thrilled to share their knowledge with you.

I am not a dedicated menopause account. I am, rather, a dedicated to shamelessness account. The most popular essay on menopause that I've written for my newsletter FEMINIST GIANT is called 'Moisturize Your Vagina'. For too long, the menopause transition has been surrounded by shame and silence. Silence fuels shame. Shame perpetuates silence. Patriarchy deploys shame like a drone: it shadows you, ready to take you out any minute, exhausting you by keeping you forever aware of its presence, to the detriment of all other things that you could be investing your attention in. I am learning, much to my thrill and awe, that one of the greatest gifts of the transition known as menopause is shamelessness. I am not known as one easily shamed, nor is modesty one of my virtues. Still, I gasp at the heights of audacity that I like to think come monthly in lieu of my menstrual cycle. It is as if, instead of shedding the lining of my uterus, I am shedding the lining of patriarchal fuckery that I was socialised into.

I am also learning to unbecome. I don't remember what I used to be and I don't know who I am becoming. But I welcome her! I have been turning, fading, swirling, coming into focus and oops-there-I-blur again as menopause kicks my fucking ass. It has been a great churner, menopause has, discombobulating all of me. It has taken whatever Mona I used to be and shaken her free at the seams. We are not taught to unbecome. And we rarely learn to unlearn or that unlearning is wreckage – of patriarchy's dicta as if smashing idols, of milestones as if shredding corsets, of 'success' that holds your ambition hostage when your anarchist heart knows it should set you free.

Menopause is shit. Menopause is amazing.

I worry sometimes when I say stuff like that. I come from a generation of cis women who were socialised to leave everything that made us cis women at home, under the mattress, in the bathroom cabinet, somewhere not too obvious, so that we could 'make it' in the cis men's world. Because if those things began to poke out from underneath the mattress, spill out from the bathroom cabinet, or become so obvious that they signalled we were not cis men, then we were not up to the privilege of being allowed entry into that cis men's world, let alone 'succeed' in it.

For nonbinary, transmasc and gender-expansive people going through menopause, the transition is often compounded and further complicated by the silence and bigotry that renders their menopausal experience truly invisible.

They are not invisible; bigotry has rendered their experience invisible.

Transphobes and 'gender critical' types get upside down bananas when those of us who insist on being trans-inclusive and who recognise a gender-expansive world use phrases like 'those of us who are non-men'. That phrase accurately captures what it's like for so many of us who make it through the world at a distinct disadvantage because we are not cis men – specifically able-bodied, wealthy, cisgender heterosexual, white men.

And then everything starts to spill out. Because menopause is shit and menopause is amazing; it is a great wrecker.

'How can I compete with men when I can't sleep?'

When I read that quote in a Canadian newspaper from a perimenopausal woman who was struggling in a corporate world that was built by (able-bodied, wealthy, cisgender heterosexual, white) men for (able-bodied, wealthy, cisgender heterosexual, white) men, I knew that smashing and shredding and wrecking were the way.

We were never meant to thrive in this world built by (able-bodied, wealthy, cisgender heterosexual, white) men for (able-bodied, wealthy, cisgender heterosexual, white) men. 'How can I compete with men when I can't sleep?' The simple answer of course is you cannot. You never were meant to. That's exactly the whole fucking point of it.

So, wreck it all.

It is exactly when the once-whispered moves into the mainstream that it most matters who is speaking the once-unsaid and who continues to be sidelined and silenced. As a feminist of colour who often must write what she has long wanted to read, I know what it's like to rarely see yourself during those 'moments', 'waves' and 'movements' – words that are now being used in mainstream media to describe the greater ubiquity of menopause. Too often when feminism takes that brave dive into the deep end of a taboo, it takes along just a select few: white, wealthy, cisgender, heterosexual, able-bodied women.

Bloody Hell! is the antidote.

If you have ever menstruated, you can go through menopause, a point in life that marks twelve months without a menstrual cycle. Once you've reached the point of twelve months without a menstrual cycle, you are postmenopausal.

It is not just cis women who experience menopause. Non-binary people, trans men and other gender non-conforming groups also experience menopause and do so under even greater levels of silence and taboo. This anthology aims to expand the Menopause Moment/Wave/Movement beyond white and cis women. And also, beyond merely the 'symptoms'. This is not a medical textbook, nor a guide on how to 'remedy' or 'fix' anything. Rather, it is a collection of menopausal people, each with their own entry point into that transition. There are as many menopause stories as people who have experienced menopause, and this anthology showcases seventeen of them. And we need every story.

What if menopause is a dive into the self to explore the myths of what we're supposed to be at this stage of our life, what 'success' is, what 'milestones' to celebrate or regret? And to then wreck them. A necessary wreckage.

Use this anthology as a sledgehammer and wreck it all.

Menopause is the hardest thing that has ever happened to me. And it's the best thing I've ever gone through. Our anthology begins and ends with an invocation and a celebration of freedom.

Use this anthology as a lighthouse, guiding you towards and welcoming whoever you are becoming.

The Menopause: When We Are Free

Marilyn Muthoni Kamuru

NARRATIVES OF THE MENOPAUSE TRANSITION

When we are free, what will we do with our freedom?

Almost two decades ago, when my aunt was in her fifties, she decided to move to America. She had always lived in Kenya. A few years before, she had retired from her job, where she had been making a comfortable living. She was still married and all of her children had left home. My aunt's decision wasn't particularly unusual. Families and communities around the continent have similar stories of women who left in their forties, fifties and even sixties. An exodus of African women departing for Europe and the United States. Often this happened after the marriage of a child, or the birth of a grandchild. Yes, these women were interested in economic opportunities, but there was something else driving them. There were aunties leaving to attend a wedding or grandmothers going on the pretext of helping the new mother and ensuring the grandchild ate the 'proper food' and spoke a few words of Kikuyu, Kisii or Kiswahili. Just a visit. Some of these aunties and grandmothers were going abroad for the first time, others had visited before, but what we didn't know at the time of their departure is that this time they wouldn't be coming back. I am not sure they all knew it either.

I am about the age my aunt was when she moved to the US almost twenty years ago. When I was discussing this phenomenon with my girlfriends, we spoke about these as silent divorces, about women escaping, in a socially acceptable way, their unhappy or unsatisfactory familial situations. Women whose age and socialisation wouldn't allow them to get a divorce. And maybe some of that is true, but I don't think it is the whole truth. I don't think women are running away as much as they are running *to*.

Women in the menopause transition are encouraged to think of ourselves as socially useless, used up. But it is what women are doing with this social irrelevance that is threatening the patriarchy. The women who travel abroad are a subset of the women who in social irrelevance find permission and freedom to be. In the social irrelevance that is supposed to accompany women when they stop bearing children, women have found opportunities to feel their own desires and to create their own relevance without reference to societal expectations. Less making lemonade with lemons, and more pass the tequila and salt. The narrative most of these women have of the menopause transition isn't one that is dominated by the patriarchy's position on the value of women in the menopause, nor by their menopausal symptoms. As Dr Jen Gunter aptly states in her book *The Menopause Manifesto: Own Your Health with Facts and Feminism*, 'What the patriarchy thinks of menopause is irrelevant. Men do not get to define the value of women at any age.'[1] Instead, the narrative that seems to prevail among these African aunties is of a more feminist menopause, a phase of life that is fundamentally about freedom – women's freedom. Freedom from and, more importantly, freedom to. This narrative of the menopause transition is particularly problematic for the patriarchy.

What we are witnessing with the exodus of African women abroad in their late forties and fifties is an expression of this narrative of the menopause as freedom.

So much of what we are encouraged to focus on with the menopause transition is what ceases, what stops happening. The loudest menopause narratives are about who we stop being – women who can reproduce. The cessation of menstrual periods and the end of the reproductive phase. It is the biology of menopause and the resulting societal implications that we are encouraged to focus on. Indeed, even the purpose of menopause is explained by its evolutionary benefit to others, from the 'mother hypothesis', which holds that older mothers benefit more from investing in their current children rather than in continuing to reproduce themselves, to the 'grandmother hypothesis', which argues that grandmothers have a benefit to the reproductive success of their children and improve the survival and wellbeing of their grandchildren.[2] What doesn't seem to get anywhere near as much attention is *what is the meaning of the menopause* for women. In other words, what does it mean for a woman to live through perimenopause, menopause and into postmenopause? What do these phases (which for this piece I will refer to broadly as the menopause or the menopause transition) mean for *her life*? For our lives? What continues flowing? Somehow, even in this uniquely female life process – and it is a process, not an event – women and women's lives have become incidental. While recognising that it is all people with ovaries who experience menopause, I will use the term 'women' in this piece because I am more concerned with the gendered social and societal implications of the menopause transition as opposed to the physical biological process.

WHAT IS THE FUNCTION OF MENOPAUSE?

In my research for this piece I came across an article in *Scientific American* entitled 'The Origin of Menopause: Why Do Women Outlive Fertility?'[3] It is easy to dismiss this as a provocative title to draw in the reader, but I think it is much more than that. I think this article captures the prevalent approach to menopause while also betraying the predominant patriarchal bias in much of the work on menopause, which is the patriarchal premise that women's primary purpose is social – that women exist for reproduction and to provide care for others. In a *Nautilus* article the author states, 'Part of the mystery of menopause is that it occurs when women still likely have several decades of generally healthy life ahead of them.'[4] Essentially, the predominant framing in explaining the evolutionary role of menopause is to question the purpose of women's existence beyond reproduction. A feminist approach to menopause starts with rejecting the patriarchal insistence on centring maleness in all aspects of enquiry. And it is centring maleness that generates this type of query, because the question is forcing women's post-reproductive existence into a question while implicitly normalising men's ability to remain fertile until close to the end of their lives.

Perhaps the fact that women continue to live beyond their reproductive life and the fact that the default foetal condition is an ovary (it is the presence of the Y chromosome that prompts development of testicles)[5] are evidence of a more female-centred evolutionary model than we have previously considered.

A feminist evolutionary approach would never think to ask why women live past their reproductive utility. A feminist approach would be satisfied with women's existence: women exist to exist. What if the point of menopause is women's being? Freedom. That women get to be themselves for THEMSELVES without purpose for OTHERS. What if the revolutionary *evolutionary* purpose of menopause is women's freedom? One of the things that has struck me about older women in the later stages of the menopause transition is their enthusiasm and excitement whenever we discuss the menopause transition. Yes, we gripe about the hot flashes and laugh about the mood swings, but without fail, every single one of these women, be they employees, entrepreneurs, married, divorced, separated or never married, has told me that this is the best stage of their lives, that they feel more confident in who they are, more satisfied with their bodies and themselves. More free.

So much of the attention on menopause is on the unpleasant physical manifestations – the irritability, mood swings, hot flashes (and I don't mean to minimise them; I am writing through some of the most intense hot flashes now) – and not enough on the power and possibility of this time for women. Add to this the medicalised and pathologised model of menopause, which treats the menopause as a disease to be managed – an aberration or deviation from the norm thrusting women into the background, reducing us to our symptoms. This medicalisation of menopause, particularly prominent in the global north/global minority but being aggressively exported around the world, reduces women to medical subjects, and in so doing emphasises all the ways in which women can be 'fixed'. And fixing is at cost, resulting in the increasing commercialisation of menopause. This isn't an argument against the treatment of menopause symptoms; rather, it is an attempt to distinguish between narratives that *equate* women to their menopause symptoms and ones that recognise physical symptoms of menopause as only one aspect of a more complicated process, one that is biological but also social and cultural.

MODERN MENOPAUSE

At the same time as our African aunties are choosing to cross continents, we are witnessing other African aunties, in the menopausal transition, reach for some of their most career-transgressive and ambitious public roles. Ellen Johnson Sirleaf was fifty-nine when she first ran for president and sixty-seven when she was elected President of Liberia. Joyce Banda was sixty-two when she was elected President of Malawi, and Samia Suluhu Hassan was sixty-one when she assumed the presidency of Tanzania. In Kenya, Charity Ngilu and Professor Wangarĩ Maathai were the first two women to vie for president in 1997, and they were forty-five and fifty-seven years old respectively. In 2021 Kenya got its first woman Chief Justice; at the time of her appointment, Martha Koome was sixty-one years old. Martha Karua, the first female deputy presidential candidate of a leading political party in Kenya, was fifty-six when she unsuccessfully ran for the presidency in 2013. In 2004, at the age of sixty-four, Professor Wangarī Maathai was awarded the Nobel Peace Prize. And seven years later, in 2011, the same prize was jointly awarded to President Ellen Johnson Sirleaf, then seventy-three, and fellow Liberian Leymah Gbowee, thirty-eight.

The experiences of these African women, from aunties to presidents and Nobel Prize laureates, are manifestations of the power of the menopause-transition narrative. Yes, they are a result of the opportunities now available to women, but *which* opportunities women seize is dependent on the menopause narrative they adopt.

For many African women, the menopause transition is a time of freedom. A time when patriarchy no longer cares, when it is focused on the women in their pre-reproductive and reproductive stages, and then we are free. In their chapter 'Normality, Freedom, and Distress: Listening to the Menopausal Experiences of Indian Women of Haryana', Dr Vanita Singh and Professor M. Sivakami remind us that: 'It is important to understand the meanings of menopause as constructed by women themselves as an alternative to overreliance on the medical discourse.' Their chapter in *The Palgrave Handbook of Critical Menstruation Studies* provides further evidence of how the narratives of the menopause transition affect the meaning of menopause for women, and of the importance of allowing women's experiences to exist in greater complexity. They found 'three distinct but co-occurring narratives that emerged were: menopause as a normal life transition, menopause as distress because it's taboo, and menopause as freedom from monthly distress and societal restrictions'.[6] In contrast to the disempowering 'medicalisation of menopause' and 'commercialisation of menopause' narratives, these global south/global majority narratives evident in the experiences of a subset of African and Indian women offer empowering and more expansive narratives of the menopause.

Why is this important? Because the power of narratives cannot be underestimated. Narratives are one of the most powerful ways in which we embody and transmit ideology, and as feminist Srilatha Batliwala reminds us in *All About Power: Understanding Social Power and Power Structures*, 'Ideology is the most powerful tool created to protect a power structure, because it is the mechanism through which everyone is convinced to participate in that oppressive system, rather than toppling it – they are taught to accept their place in society.'[7] Narratives that recognise the complexity of the menopause transition and how it can manifest differently for different women based on a multiplicity of factors are necessary to ensuring women have more individual and social power during this period. This is especially important as the predominant global minority narratives are narrower and significantly less empowering for women. This divergence in global south/global majority and global north/global minority approaches to the menopause is also important because it has implications well beyond menopause. On average, women in Africa will spend about a third of their lives in the menopause transition[8] and in East Asia women will spend a quarter of their lives.[9] And according to the World Health Organization, this demographic is growing: 'In 2021, women aged 50 and over accounted for 26 per cent of all women and girls globally.'[10] More than a quarter of the girls and women alive are in the menopause transition. This is a significant portion of the global adult population, and the increased social, economic and political power of this demographic, in addition to its size, poses unprecedented challenges and opportunities for societies across the globe.

POWER AND VULNERABILITY

Unsurprisingly, patriarchy's response to narratives that result in women's expanded freedom during the menopause is violent. It is to try to crush women and put them back in 'their place', to force women away from being the main characters in their own stories. Patriarchy's response is to try to put down the insurrection that is the menopause.

As such, at the same time that African women adopt this 'menopause as freedom' narrative, and as women age within the menopause, there is an escalation in women's vulnerability. In this way the menopause remains a stage where women continue to exist at risk of patriarchal violence: physical, sexual, economic and psychological. While disappointing, it isn't surprising, because it follows a familiar pattern in patriarchal societies: as women acquire power, they often become targets for violence. For African women, the social irrelevance that is supposed to accompany this phase is a form of liberation from societal norms and strictures, but with this liberation, older women model a form of female freedom that is threatening to the patriarchal establishment in ways that make them socially relevant again.

According to the World Economic Forum, no woman alive today will experience gender parity in her lifetime.[11]

However, women have more legal, economic and political rights than they have had at any other time in history, and because of the sheer number of women in the menopause transition globally, as well as the developments in media, from the internet to community radio, that have enabled access to more information, especially peer to peer, the menopause transition is increasingly posing an existential threat to patriarchy.

This is important because the reason women in the menopause transition become socially relevant again is that their existence itself is perceived as a problem. According to Leo Igwe of Advocacy for Alleged Witches in West Africa, 'Witchcraft accusations have a female face in Africa.' And while there has been and continues to be significant work around the violence faced by mostly older women in Africa targeted as witches, what has not been made explicit is their connection with this phase of the menopause transition. Across the continent, the women overwhelmingly isolated and targeted for violence as witches are older and elderly women, many of them widows. Yet these articles and organisations working on witch-hunting rarely make the connection between the menopause transition and the isolation, targeting and violence against older and elderly women. Even when the pattern is there for all to see between women, widows and alleged witches. Speaking about a spate of murders of women accused of witchcraft in Kenya in 2021, Carole Osero-Ageng'o of HelpAge International stated that: 'Most of the victims are widows whose accusers are relatives from families of their deceased husbands. Witchcraft accusations are traceable to land scarcity, greed, selfishness, and misogyny.'[12] Reliable data on witchcraft allegations and attacks against older women is not readily available.[13] In Tanzania, where witchcraft allegations and the killing of women accused of witchcraft is a serious concern, Helen Kijo-Bisimba, executive director of Tanzania's Legal and Human Rights Centre, tells us that the reason is land. She goes on to state, '[The Widows] are supposed to bequeath it when they die – and they don't die.'[14] Which harkens back to the title of the *Scientific American* article, 'Why Do Women Outlive Fertility?' In other words, why don't women die when we stop being useful to men?

So often the preoccupation is with deconstructing, delegitimising or rubbishing witchcraft, such that there is no serious reflection on what it is that witchcraft and the label of witches are masking. If we ignore the question of the validity of a belief in witchcraft, what could be behind this particular form of violence against women by men – VAWBM* (and it is predominantly men)? Patriarchy isn't a rational system, but it is a highly adaptive system. It morphs, it adjusts; this is how it survives. Therefore, witchcraft can be a belief of a patriarchal system to address the fear embodied by the existence of older and elderly women, especially widows who live in ways that model and normalise female freedom that is otherwise not permitted in these societies. Women living unattached and unanswerable to men, especially older men. Especially as their numbers continue to grow. Women with control of resources (inheritance of land, animals, etc.) all threaten a society that has male dominance and male control of resources as an organising tenet. What is important, then,

---

* I use this term instead of the more common VAW because it names the perpetrator of the violence, returning the perpetrators of the violence to the frame.

is to address what this belief seeks to do, what purpose it serves in the society. This belief is rooted in patriarchy and seeks to reassert the power and dominance of men and their control of resources through all stages of women's lives.

Widows, especially, are then both powerful and vulnerable at the same time. But this duality of power and vulnerability isn't restricted to widows. It is at the crux of the menopause transition for all women: the control of resources, which includes our bodies but also our choices and narratives. With the 'medicalisation of menopause' and increasingly the 'commercialisation of menopause' the common denominator seems to be to distract women from the real potential of this phase – the power and promise of the menopause transition – by focusing on the symptoms of menopause, the deficiencies of women, and how they can, through the purchase of supplements, hormones, fans and smartwatches, be magically 'fixed'. Amplifying the vulnerabilities of the menopause transition is to prime women to adopt narratives that promote a patriarchal ideology. Complicating the menopause transition is important to expanding women's freedom during this period, and it requires an understanding of both the possibilities as well as vulnerabilities of this phase.

As part of the feminist project, I am interested in exploring and amplifying narratives that expand women's power to give women in different spaces and stages an opportunity to live in more expansive ways. As such, I am drawn to narratives that expand possibilities for women and repelled by those that are based on a belief that women are deviant or inherently pathological.

CONCLUSION

Menopause as a phase is probably the most powerful time in a woman's life because it challenges the patriarchal paradigm. So women need to ask themselves: what do I do with my power? How do I enter and experience this phase? Maybe you will deepen your engagement in your chosen area of expertise like President Ellen Johnson Sirleaf or Chief Justice Martha Koome, or you will go out into the world to explore like our aunties, or you will help in the raising of your grandchildren, or build your dream home in the village or finally write that book or books. The menopause transition isn't a caterpillar or butterfly phase – it is both. There are lifetimes in the menopause transition. This is an individual but also a collective liberation. The greater freedom each individual woman has, the more freedom expands for women generally, and therein lies both power and danger. This is especially important in this moment as we witness the global increase in the number of women in the menopause transition.

When we live in ways that defy patriarchal paradigms, we expand the possibilities for ourselves and each other. As such, while our individual freedom as women is important, the acceptance and adoption of more expansive narratives of the menopause transition have the effect of offering collective freedom for us as women. What continues to flow is so much more important than what ceases in the menopause transition. Whatever you do when you enter the menopause transition, allow yourself to flow, to meander, to be in this phase just like a river is. Allow yourself the experience of the rapids, especially for those of us with more severe symptoms of the menopause and those of us experiencing difficult life events, from deaths to care of ageing parents. Revel in the stillness that comes with increasing social irrelevance, the possibilities of freedom that come from existing for ourselves, by ourselves: you will not drown. Water cannot drown. The most important and urgent question of the menopause transition is what will we do with our freedom?

Marilyn Muthoni Kamuru (she/her) is a feminist lawyer, political strategist and policy advisor based in Kenya. She holds a BA in political science from Northeastern University and a JD (Juris Doctor) and LLM (Master of Laws) in international and comparative law from Cornell Law School. Her writing has appeared in *The Elephant*, Al Jazeera, *Foreign Policy*, *Politics & Gender*, *Daily Nation*, *The Standard* and *Business Daily*. In 2021 she was named one of the 100 Most Influential People in Gender Policy by Apolitical (apolitical.co).

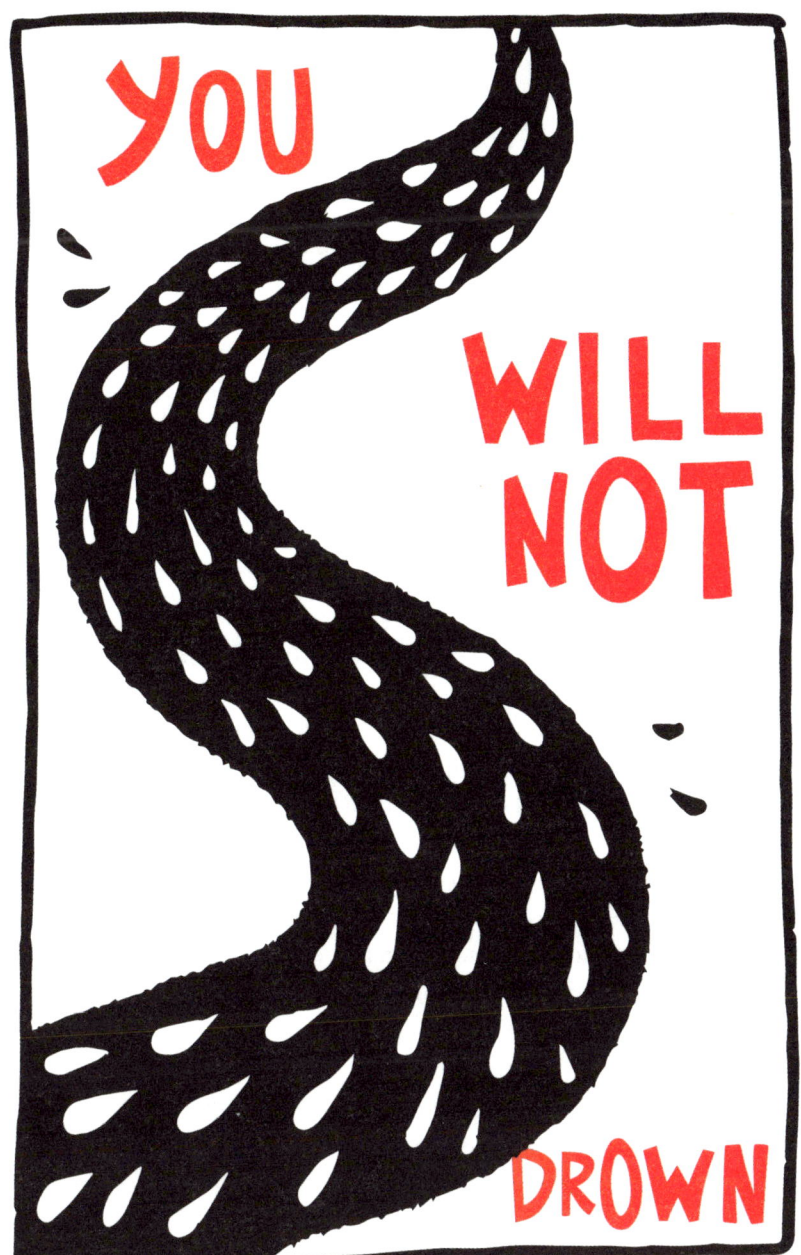

The Yellies

Simi Hoque

'I want Papa.'
'Why?'
'Because he doesn't yell at us.'

I have the *yellies*. I have them All The Time between 6 p.m. and 10 p.m., during the only real close family time that I have with my three children and when my partner is still at work teaching courses at the university. It's gotten worse, and at first I suspected quarantine fatigue. In March 2020, my children came home from school and didn't leave me alone for the next sixteen months. We all started working from home, carving out space in basements, closets, bedrooms and kitchens, and I began accumulating rage, grief, anxiety and overwhelm. I started sweatily catastrophising at 2 a.m. every night. Intimacy fled, hugs were scarce. My concentration and memory fractured. Reading about real life and humans was impossible; dragons and aliens became my friends. My colleagues gently told me that I lacked composure. To which I wanted to yell, 'I've been sipping on toxic masculinity for four decades now – what did you expect?!' I thought that being promoted to full professor would mean that I would have a better handle on being a woman in a male-dominated field, that the imposter symptoms would finally fade, that with age came a gravitas that meant I wouldn't get talked over. Instead, I felt more insecure, anxious and destabilised. It was like I was going through puberty all over again.

I started gaining belly fat in more places than my abdomen. Going to the gym was a non-starter – those tiny, tight, thirty-year-old athletes made me feel old, fat and weak. I used to play tennis and loved the camaraderie of joint exertion, but now I just couldn't find people my age who weren't too busy or broken to play. I bought a spin bike, treadmill and a Peloton subscription. I started running and signed up for road races. Over time, I got closer to the podium. Not because I was any faster or stronger, but because there were fewer women my age doing these things. I gritted my teeth through joint aches and kept trying. I got hurt more frequently. I had to take multiple rest days. Going for a run required a lot of planning because I had to spend as much time stretching and foam rolling as I had on the run itself. Working out and running was lonely. I tried group classes like CrossFit, Pure Barre and Orange Theory. But the studios were filled with people who looked like my students, fresh and feisty, not achy and angsty like me.

I found inspiration for my aspirational goals among a subculture of older athletes on YouTube who emphasised doing less cardio and more strength training. All the aerobic exercise that I was doing was actually causing more stress on my body, leading to more weight gain rather than loss. But the only way I could get free of my head was to do really hard things at a high intensity. How was I to balance the immediate relief of tempo workouts against the long-term cortisol increases that it led to? A friend told me about a book she was reading by exercise physiologist and nutrition scientist Dr Stacy Sims and pro-cyclist Selene Yeager called *Next Level* that focused on older female athletes. Women my age need to incorporate strength training because muscle loss becomes more pronounced as oestrogen levels decrease. The decline in muscle mass had started in my thirties, but it was now accelerating because getting old sucks more if you're weak and can't lift heavy things. But none of my friends wanted to lift weights: there is a persistent myth that lifting would make us hulky-bulky. I was willing to accept a little bulk to avoid getting hurt, but I did not want to put in the time to become a powerlifter. There did not appear to be an in-between. I tried to develop my own resistance-training programme, focusing specifically on the muscles that I needed to strengthen for mobility, for balance, for endurance, and to deadlift my ninety-year-old father when he fell, which was distressingly more often.

Meanwhile, my hair was thinning and my skin felt papery. My face broke out. And even though I was using all the filters on Zoom, my own face did not please me any more. I bought makeup and looked up Instagram tutorials for people who don't wear makeup. I discovered a mature lady on Instagram who explained how to hide my drooping eyelids. I didn't even know that I had this affliction until I saw the video. A friend showed me her magnifying mirror and I realised that my age-induced farsightedness was actually a blessing. Why buy this mirror when it makes me feel bad? Ah, because

I cannot see how poorly I'm applying eyeliner any more. A dermatologist I talked to said that I had 'maskne'*, but I did not mask so much, since I was working from home. She gave me a prescription for retinol and had a cosmetic dermatologist talk to me about treatments for wrinkles and age spots. Why is it so hard to accept the natural process? I did not want to pay for Botox, laser therapy or chemical peels. I just didn't want to look like a hormonal teen. I read about taking collagen supplements – that they would help restore my skin's firmness and moisture, but I got a gruesome stomach-ache and ridiculously hard nails instead.

I changed my diet, saying goodbye to Goldfish crackers (processed), Quadratini wafers (sugar) and French fries (grease). My best friend told me that very few people are getting enough fibre, and that blended green smoothies were not adequate. I started eating Ezekiel 4:9's whole-grains-and-gravel-in-a-box cereal for breakfast. Further research indicated that I was also not getting enough protein, so I replaced Oreos with boiled eggs and Greek yogurt for my snack. But my skin still looked tired, and I was chronically exhausted. After learning from Matthew Walker's *Why We Sleep* that drinking alcohol in the evening affects our sleep, I resorted to daytime drinking and perfected a sublime margarita before 3 p.m. Then I learned to avoid caffeine and alcohol altogether and sleep in a cold room. I wondered whether all these changes would only make me more boring, not better rested with more supple skin. I saw a board-certified medical doctor who was also an acupuncturist. She told me about adaptogens, plant-based

---

* Acne breakouts caused by wearing a face mask.

supplements to manage my stress and fatigue. She recommended *Schisandra* to improve my endurance and *Rhodiola* to reduce pain and fatigue. I was coming full circle – my people had been drinking tulsi tea and taking ashwagandha as an ayurvedic therapy for decades. Conventional Western medicine was finally giving some space for South Asian knowledge. Yet nothing really seemed to be helping – the massive changes that I made to my diet, exercise and sleep did little to ease the angst, rage and sense that something was wrong.

I was furiously stronger, fitter and eating better. I bought an Oura Ring to track how well I was sleeping. The ring was supposed to learn from me, but my sleep was so erratic and problematic that it felt like she (the algorithm) was chiding me every morning: 'Suboptimal sleep patterns, consider reviewing your pre-sleep routine, stress and activity level.' If I listened to the recommendations from the ring, every day would be a rest day and I would have to go to sleep by 9 p.m. Who does that? I did. I actually made an effort to go to bed at 9 p.m, even before my teenage kids, but I invariably woke up at 2 a.m. with restless legs and deep anxiety. I started talking to a therapist and she offered me a framework to make sense of my moods – it is called Internal Family Systems. It was a way to see myself as a combination of many parts that were sometimes dysregulated. My anxiety was a part of me, just as my malice and frustration were. These were not bad parts, just guests in my house, and I could look to them as guides from beyond. What were these guides telling me? Was the problem something that I was or was not doing? Was this part of what American doctor John Sarno called the mind-body connection? Was I sublimating my emotions into my body? Was that what was creating all the emotional and physical turbulence?

I was angry all the time, and everything was not awesome. I took a workshop in non-violent communication so that I would not shame my children for things that I was aggravated about. At work, my students needed more time and more grace than I was able to find within myself. How could I learn to speak with compassion when there was so much noise in my head? Is this a condition of the modern age? When did I become so overscheduled? My sister told me to stop trying to do so much. I started quitting things to reduce my load. No more board membership. No more associate editor. No more service committees. No more conference presentations. No more panels. No more advisory roles. I reached my limit, and it was time for my Great Resignation. I left everything except what really mattered to me and what would keep me employed. I had been carrying around an idea of my importance, that I was needed in all these different ways. Quitting was a wake-up call about how unnecessarily busy I had been.

This is freedom, I thought. But it was also something else. I was also realising that the rate at which my invisibility was spreading was not equal to the rate of my not giving a fuck. How do women in their forties cope with this? Do men have these issues? My parents were getting older much faster, and my kids were not getting older fast enough. I felt like Chewbacca in the trash compactor, being crushed from both sides with a carnivorous monster in my head. I was now squarely in the 'sandwich generation', witnessing the decline of my parents, trying to balance their care, while also not neglecting the growth and emotional resilience of my coming-of-age teens.

Did this count as a midlife crisis? Was I crazy? All my friends clamoured, 'SAME!' Except, when pandemic-related shit started settling down, they found equilibrium, and I added forgetfulness and headaches to my list of fuckery. My work was suffering and I told my dean that I was burnt out. She sympathised. It is not easy being a woman in a STEM field, but it is even harder when you cannot remember shit because you have what looks like long Covid symptoms without even having had Covid. I did not have any models for how to manage my work and family responsibilities on top of feeling like crap. Was this a sign that being a good mother, successful professor, supportive partner and middle-of-the-pack athlete in America is asking too much? I listened to an effervescent Black medical doctor online describe Every Single Thing that I was experiencing. Apparently, I'm not crazy. I am perimenopausal, and women of colour enter the journey earlier. Forty-five is not 'too young', as my thirty-nothing-year-old white ob-gyn had told me.

I went to see a different doctor. And another. And another. They either brushed off my concerns as a 'normal part of the ageing process' or prescribed medications that did not seem like they addressed the root cause of the symptoms I was experiencing. We are all led to believe that our lives are basically over and we will become obsolete at menopause. There are so many myths around this journey. I waded through many of them. No, I do not want antidepressants. No, I do not want sleeping pills. No, steroids will only work for a short time and twelve weeks of physical therapy doesn't seem to be helping. I was unwilling to stop running and lifting heavy weights. Not one of the doctors I went to brought up the topic of menopause, and my own research and self-discovery process yielded far more robust solutions than those that they offered. Why didn't anyone tell me what was going to happen to my mind and body? Why is this a big secret? If half the human race will spend just about half their lives in menopause, why are doctors so reluctant to talk or ignorant about this?

My doctor friends could not remember learning about menopause in medical school. The miseducation of doctors can be traced to the Women's Health Initiative (WHI), a US study that was stalled in the early 2000s and led to the elimination of menopause education in medical schools. The WHI's preliminary findings showed a small increase in risk of heart disease and breast cancer from hormone therapy (HT), thereby removing the only solution to menopause that doctors had learned about. Now that HT had a bad rap, big medicine no longer wanted to touch it or fund research for alternative solutions.

The diversity of symptoms, both physical and emotional, that women go through during this phase is mind-boggling. Hormone therapy is but one of multiple strategies that women going through menopause symptoms might adopt. I tried to find a certified menopause practitioner who could explain the pros and cons of the things I was teaching myself about – adaptogens, breath work, cherry juice, cognitive behaviour therapy, microdosing, meditation, yoga and hormone therapy – but the calculus of finding a person who lived in my area, who carried my insurance, who was taking new patients, who would listen to me ... it took time that my doctors did not have to wade through all the intricacies, and I am not a patient person. I wanted to stop inopportunely sweating so robustly, to be able to sleep through the night, to stop being aggravated that everyone was stupid or difficult, to remember why I had come upstairs to begin with, to not feel like I was working all the time and out of time.

It has been three years since I started feeling crazy. I'm still grappling with it, but now I have named it, acknowledged that it's happening, and meditated the hell out of my 2 a.m. catastrophes. Nothing has really changed. I am still not reading about real people and real things, but I can now credit that to the M-word, as well as the general shit state of this planet, dismal diversity in STEM, having teenage children, school start times, climate change, ageing parents and that I never want to wear hard pants* again. Like most things, menopause is intersectional, and I really cannot attribute my symptoms of malaise and pain to just one thing. There are multiple pathways and imperfect solutions. I can take HT, eat soy and take fish oil. I can eat a plant-based diet, avoid alcohol and caffeine, focus on fibre and exercise daily. I can cultivate friendships, take art classes and volunteer regularly. All these strategies might lead to relief, or they might not. The important thing, for me, is that I am no longer flapping my hands helplessly and haplessly. I know enough about perimenopause and its symptoms to address them using a toolkit of strategies. The past two years have been educational, drawing from the shared wisdom of perimenopausal women in my circle of friends as well as from the growing list of athletes, doctors, institutions and researchers that speak and write about this online.

I am delighted that more and more women are speaking about hormones and menopause; it is now in the zeitgeist because people like Oprah and Michelle Obama have talked

---

* An informal term for types of trousers with zips, buttons or non-elasticated waists that are less comfortable than those primarily worn or designed for comfort.

about their struggles with it. Most women who go through perimenopause will experience some kind of systemic breakdown – brain fog, exhaustion, hot flashes, sleep disruption, weight gain, loss of libido, depression, dry skin . . . these are simply some of the many symptoms of menopause that women should be aware of. It is time to educate ourselves and our doctors about these symptoms, and to find strategies to address them that fit with our lifestyle and needs. I have read papers from the National Institutes of Health, Cleveland and Mayo Clinics, WebMD, Healthline and the North American Menopause Society for information. I have also listened to the podcasts *Hit Play Not Pause*, *Menopause Management with Menopause Barbie*, *The Dr Louise Newson Podcast* and *With All Due Respect*. And I have tried many different types of therapies, from acupuncture to EMDR (eye movement desensitisation and reprocessing). I still run (probably too much) and lift heavy weights. But I have convinced enough friends to join me in getting stronger and more resilient as we navigate this new chapter.

I know that I am not alone – half of the world's population will go through menopause – so we should talk about this with each other, our partners, daughters and sons openly, factually and unabashedly. When I first started talking about my symptoms – after I learned what it was – I was very hesitant to name it. Somehow it felt like I was talking about something really private and personal, something that would stigmatise me as a woman. But then I realised that this was part of the problem – that my younger female friends would all go through this cycle of feeling cray-cray if they didn't hear about perimenopause explicitly from people who were going through it. So now I'm working towards normalising it for what it is – a life transition that affects all of us one way or another. There are days that I feel almost normal, giddy with the idea that I am finally not scared. I am only just getting started, because what other people think will not stop me from being me. It is such a relief to just leave when I want. To be on the road towards not giving a fuck and reaching for what I want. Everything that I have leaned in and worked towards for the past forty-eight years has been a glorious prelude to this next chapter of my story, the one that I get to tell now, with more humour and honesty than before.

Simi Hoque (she/her) is a professor of architectural engineering at Drexel University whose research focuses on sustainability and wellbeing in buildings. She is a Bangladeshi American academic who juggles motherhood, triathlon training and a deep love of reading with her need to get enough sleep and have a good life.

LIKE MOST THINGS

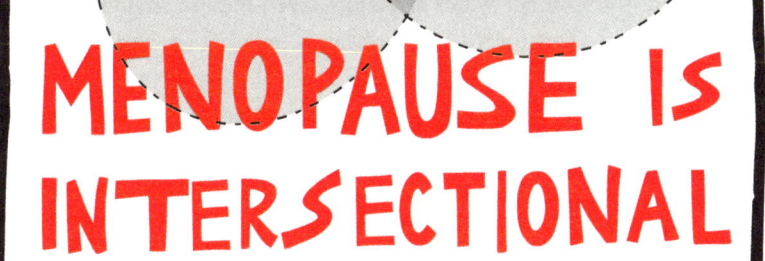

MENOPAUSE IS INTERSECTIONAL

Bits of Flesh: For Anarcha – From Enslavement to Menopause

Omisade Burney-Scott

Anarcha sat on the cold hard table with her knees tucked under her skirts. Her blouse was unbuttoned to her navel, exposing her breasts, her chin up and firmly set as her eyes searched for a spot on the wall, her spot on the wall where she could focus her breath as tears formed in her eyes. Like Lucy and Betsy before her, she knew what would happen next. Her long dark brown fingers gathered her skirt in bunches, she steadied herself for the pain that she would experience – sometimes dull but, more often than not, searing and unrelenting as Massa Sims carved out bits of flesh from her body down there. She had stopped bleeding with the moon long ago and could not hold her water any more, even though she had not yet reached her forty-fifth birthday. Three babies had come. Some stayed with her . . . others were sold. Three more babies came but never took their first breath. Massa Sims said he could 'fix her', but after working on her several times over the year, she still urinated on herself and was punished for smelling by being sent to work in the field.

As he instructed her to 'lie down, gal' before a gallery of spectators, she thought, *My name is Anarcha, like my nanny.* She did what she was instructed to do, lying flat on her back and slowly letting her legs fall open, and for a moment, she shifted her eyes from her spot on the wall to the white faces watching. She realised they were only watching him and wondered if they could see her too. Did they see the warm salty tears running down the sides of her face as she prayed silently to herself for relief to ease her pain? Did they hear her muffled cries as Massa Sims chided, 'Hush up now, gal,' as he did his 'work' that would leave her trembling and aching in the most private areas of her body?

My people could fly

Whether they did or not, it would not change her lot. She turned her head back to focus her eyes on her spot and watched it grow. She willed her spirit to be lifted out of her body and to fly away as the Black folks did in the stories her nanny told her. She closed her eyes and prayed to the gods of her ancestors to help her. She prayed for her children and silently called the names of her ancestors to gather around her as she focused her breathing and her eyes on her spot. The tingle started in her left pinky toe and moved slowly up her leg as the sound of the crude tools scraping the platter beside the table Massa Sims used – one then another, inside and outside her private parts – started to fade. Her breath grew shallow as she realised something was happening. Her spot on the wall began to spread, and she could see outside the building.

My people could fly

She started to panic until she turned her head to look at the small group of faces still focused on Massa Sims' work and not on her. They didn't appear to see the wall disappearing or her skin beginning to glow. Anarcha closed her eyes tightly and began to moan as she felt her spirit slowly detach from her body and rise up in the gallery. When she opened her eyes, she was in the in-between place where space and time meet. She looked down and could see herself on the table, Massa Sims standing between her legs, sleeves rolled up, hands bloody, concentrating on his 'work' and the indiscernible faces of the watchers. She looked at her spot on the wall, and she now could see through it clearly, and there stood her nanny, the babies that came but didn't stay who were no longer babies, and a host of people who looked like her, smiling and waving as they hovered in the sky of pastel blues and purple. She opened her mouth to speak, but nothing came out, so she looked at Nanny and thought . . .

> It hurts
> *I know, baby . . .*
> I'm tired
> *Take my hand*
> I'm scared
> *Take my hand*
> I don't want to hurt any more
> *We can fly*
> I just wanna be free
> *You can fly*

THE MENOPAUSE LANDSCAPE

By 2025, over 1 billion people will experience menopause worldwide – 12 per cent of the world population. Though menopause is a critical point on the reproductive justice spectrum, less than 30 per cent of medical students in the USA receive substantive training on the subject. Less than 3 per cent of US ob-gyns have expertise in menopause. This is staggering, considering the number of people who are or will be menopausal and how menopausal physiological experiences are linked to increased risks of cardiovascular disease, sleep disturbances and changes in brain cognition and mood.

Generations of Black women, trans and gender-expansive people in the US have struggled to feel agency over their bodies. Since the enslavement of Africans throughout the diaspora, whiteness and the experiences of white people have been centred as the norm. Experiences outside of the norm are othered, marginalised or dehumanised. Health equity, women's health, ageing and reproductive rights for marginalised and invisibilised communities all come together in response to menopause. Resources for menopausal people have been sparse. What exists has been primarily built for individuals who identify as cisgender and heterosexual, and are likely in their forties or fifties.

White supremacy, patriarchy and misogyny all play significant roles in how the stigma of ageing and evolving women-identified bodies translate across generations. The silence is concerning and dangerous for Black, indigenous and other non-Black women, trans and gender-expansive people who experience menopause earlier and may have more prolonged and intense symptoms than their white counterparts. The sociopolitical realities of systemic oppression in the medical-industrial complex impact these experiences. Rather than being harnessed as a positive transformation with a spectrum of stages and manifestations, menopause is cloaked in fear and isolation.

The Black Girl's Guide to Surviving Menopause (BGG2SM) was created to counterbalance prevalent harmful narratives and a lack of resources. BGG2SM is a multidisciplinary initiative focused on cultural organising, narrative shift work and advocacy. Understanding the historical and contemporary experiences of Black women, trans and gender-expansive people – intergenerationally, across class and through a gender and racial equity lens – is critical for body sovereignty. We believe that Black people are the experts of our own bodies. Owning our stories is vital to having agency over our experiences, relationships and liberation. By integrating reproductive justice, radical Black feminism and gender liberation, BGG2SM normalises menopause by centring first-person narratives of those who exist at the margins of the growing menopause landscape. We nurture a community that includes all voices and lived experiences: cis, trans, intersex, queer, straight, affluent, low-wealth, activists and creatives.

An emerging menopause industry is booming, with telehealth enterprises and wellness empires. More employers are implementing menopause-friendly work policies, and menopause is now regularly covered in the media. The US Congress has even introduced the bipartisan Menopause Research Act of 2022, requiring the National Institutes of Health to conduct an evaluation of menopause-related research and identify further needed research. While all these initiatives are to be welcomed, the current landscape continues to revolve primarily around the voices, realities and influence of high-profile, affluent, cis, hetero, white women. The work they lead is monetised both by the private sector and philanthropy. Amplifying and supporting the physical, mental, spiritual and political needs of all Black people at the intersection of ageing, gender and race is sacred work and healing for our ancestral throughline.

We do this work for those navigating their menopause now, those who came before us, and those who will experience menopause in the future. In the same way, we understand that the blood memory of epigenetics carries trauma from one generation to the next; it also carries ancestral medicine, healing and love. We are the children of the people who could fly.

THE MENOPAUSAL MULTIVERSE

Approximately 40 billion Earth-size planets are orbiting habitable zones of sunlight stars and red dwarf stars within the Milky Way galaxy. One of the spiral arms of the Milky Way is called the Orion Arm. This is where our Earth is located.

We are located inside a solar system that consists of eight planets, numerous comets, asteroids and dwarf planets that orbit our sun inside a galaxy, inside of a universe that exists inside a multiverse. In the multiverses that exist, dimensions transcend length, width, depth and time. According to string theory, the multiverse operates in ten dimensions that also include:

Possible worlds
A plane of all possible worlds with the same start conditions
A plane of all possible worlds, each with different start conditions
A plane of all possible worlds starting out differently, with each branching out infinitely
All possible worlds – starting with all possible start conditions and laws of physics
And lastly,
Infinite possibilities ... EVERYTHING is possible.[1]

When Anarcha reached out to touch her nanny's hand, she realised she was hovering above the ground. She didn't feel weightless, but rather a lightness in her spirit met with a warm buzzing feeling. She could feel the wind and the sun on the back of her neck and smell honeysuckle in the air. She closed her eyes, sighed deeply, floating through the veil into the space where time bends, and felt the soft pressure of a hand on her shoulder. Anarcha moved her body to come face to face with a young woman who looked like her but was very different. The young woman wore a white button-down linen shirt tucked into wide-leg white linen pants. Large brass earrings adorned her ears, and her thick, black, coarse hair was braided with gold thread interwoven, and coiled into eight large knots on her head like a crown. Her full lips spread into a gap-toothed smile that looked like Anarcha's smile, and her fingers were long and brown like Anarcha's. She was beautiful, but more than that, she looked free. When the woman opened her mouth to speak, the edges of her silhouette expanded, and there appeared to be a multitude of women floating behind her. She said ...

I am Anarcha, your great-great-great-granddaughter. I am here with a message from the future and the past. We hold stardust in our mouths and fire in our fingertips. We have never not existed. When your mother was in Nanny's womb, I was there too. You prayed for me, and I prayed for you in the language of your great-great-great-grandmother. I came because you called for me. You called out for us. We signalled our arrival with the spot on the wall, your spot.

The young women standing as legion behind younger Anarcha said . . .

We speak your name.
We reclaimed you. The blood that carries your pain and your joy runs through our veins. We are your progeny, your joy, your healing, your legacy and your wildest dreams. We are the children of the ones that did not die.

Young Anarcha pulled her great-great-great-grandmother close, so their bodies touched as she embraced her. Anarcha could smell the honeysuckle in her hair as their heartbeats echoed each other. She closed her eyes and held on as her progeny whispered in her ear . . .

We came to tell you of your destiny, Granny Anarcha. Your destiny is to do nothing but tell the truth and be a shape-shifter in your truth-telling because sometimes you have to shape-shift to tell the truth to a multitude of people for generations to come. You are worthy of

joy, goodness, kindness, tenderness and being cherished, and not on some condition. And remember . . .
    You can fly.

And with that, the young woman kissed Anarcha's palms, placing a small cowrie shell in each, and then she kissed each eyelid as a final act of loving fealty.

Anarcha slowly opened her eyes to Massa Sims and the indiscernible faces in the gallery staring at her. She realised that she was back in her body and that she had been speaking out loud. Massa looked dumbfounded as he said, 'I'm done for now, gal. You get back to the field.' Anarcha sat up, and when she began to smooth out her skirt slowly, two small cowrie shells fell into her lap. She quickly covered them with one hand, clutching her shirt together with the other. She stood up, feeling a warmth on the back of her neck that radiated down the rest of her body. She could smell honeysuckle in the room. With her head held high, she walked out of the gallery into the stretch of land between Massa's makeshift hospital and the slave cabins. She gingerly tucked the shells into the protection bag she kept tucked into the pocket of her skirt that was full of herbs and prayers given to her by her nanny when she was a girl. When she reached the field, she looked down and realised her feet were hovering two inches above the ground.

I can fly.

Omisade Burney-Scott (she/her) is a seventh-generation Black Southern feminist, storyteller, and Reproductive justice advocate. She is also the Creator and Chief Curatorial Officer of The Black Girl's Guide to Surviving Menopause (BGG2SM), a Reproductive Justice multidisciplinary narrative and culture shift project focused on normalising menopause by centering the stories of Black women, transgender, gender-expansive people, and other marginalised groups of the Global Majority. Over the past twenty-five years, Omisade's work has been grounded in social justice movement spaces focused on the liberation of marginalized people, beginning with her own community in the areas of racial, economic, reproductive, and healing justice.

In 2023, she was selected for the Open Society Foundation's Soros Justice Fellowship to elevate the stories of formerly incarcerated and system-impacted people. Omisade has served on various nonprofit boards, including Fund for Southern Communities, Spirithouse South, Village of Wisdom, Working Films, and The Beautiful Project. She currently serves on the boards of the National Menopause Foundation and the Honey Pot Company Pulse Panel. She graduated from UNC-Chapel Hill in 1989.

Omisade resides in North Carolina and is the mother of two beautiful sons.

WE ARE THE CHILDREN

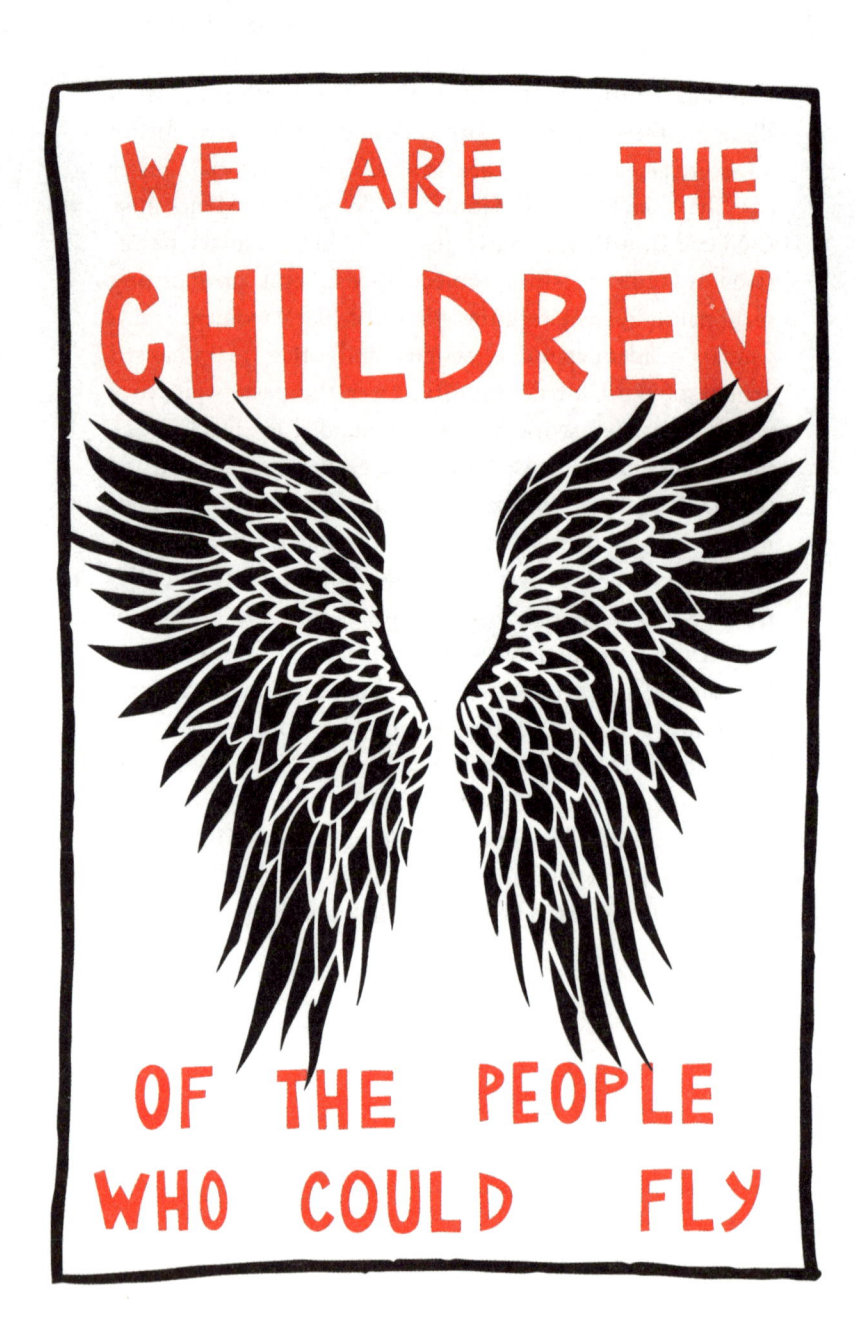

OF THE PEOPLE WHO COULD FLY

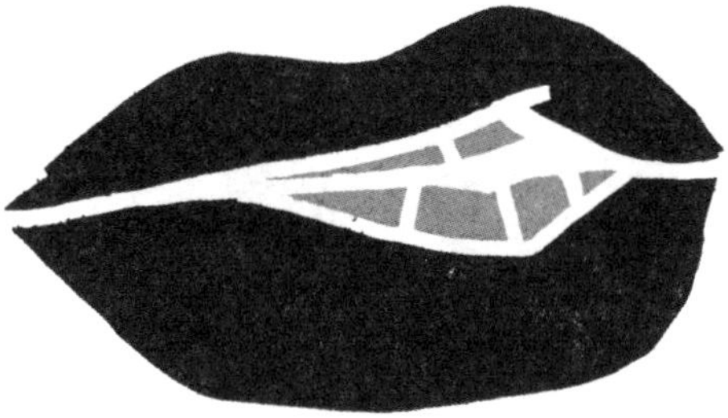

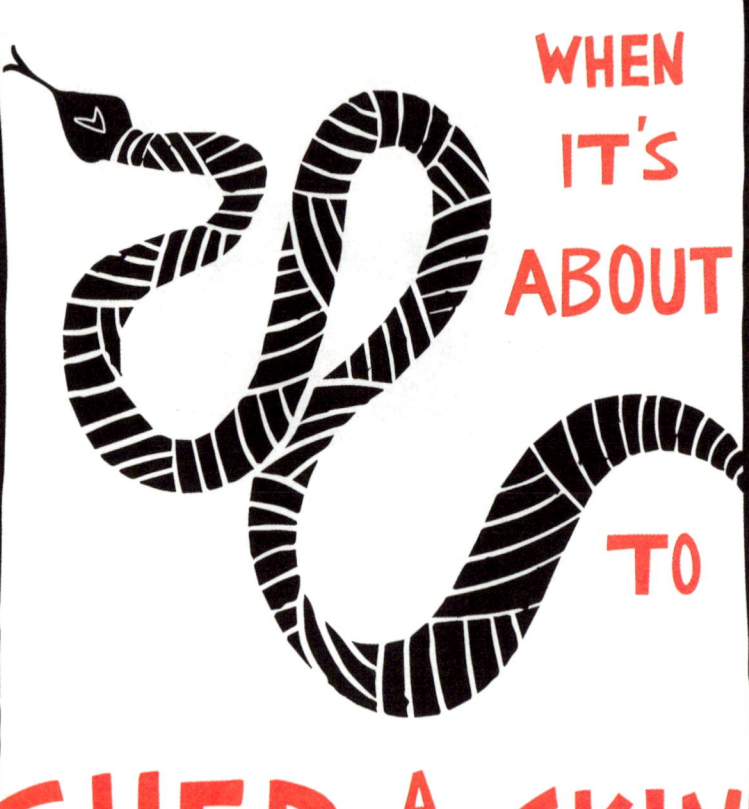

IS THIS HOW A **SNAKE FEELS** WHEN IT'S ABOUT TO **SHED A SKIN**

Gender, What Even Was That? Or, Diary of a Chest

Tania Glyde

As you move through life you are simultaneously navigating what is happening to you in the moment and the impact of your past experiences on your reactions. Your emotional mind palace is shifting constantly and you are perpetually adapting as well as creating. This process may have served you well for years.

And then along comes menopause, where the bodily changes and mood shifts feel at first like temporary ailments, then parasitic invaders, and then irrevocable morphing.

I didn't know much about menopause, even when I was bang in the middle of it. Actually, my body already knew something that I had not previously been willing, or able, to name.

THE BODY REBELS

Two years postmenopause, I discovered through a routine mammogram that I had oestrogen-receptor-positive breast cancer. From the technician's face I'd kind of guessed there was a problem. I had already had a stroke aged forty-one, and now this uncertain body had once again malfunctioned.

It's always risky to attribute symbolic value to illness, but under all the shock when I got the callback letter, something in me seemed to be released. I absolutely felt fear, but I also felt pulled into a process; a process where I just had to turn up, which felt like a luxury.

The waiting, the biopsy, more waiting, the diagnosis, more waiting, then the cutting and then the radiating. And then more waiting. I had been dragged onto the healthcare conveyer belt and, not for the first time, I felt held by it.

For a number of years up to this time, I had been looking in the mirror and, increasingly, my reflection returned nothing congruent, nothing that felt right. Medium-length hair dyed too often. Too many halfway-house clothes. None of this was working for me any more and had not, in truth, for a long time. I had kept the hair for a while partly to cover a temporary skin condition, but also to give the finger to sneery biphobia and being Not Queer Enough. Part of me did not want to change my appearance simply in order to be accepted.

Back to cancer. Wide lump excision day is a long one. It's not just one procedure but three, with a very early start. I sat and waited and then went into a giant camera machine and then waited some more and then they stuck a wire into me to point to the lump so that the surgeons could see it. This process involved submission, loss of control and acceptance. It took me back to any number of dungeons I had passed through at one time or another. (At fifteen hours in total, this experience was, it has to be said, a hell of a scene.) I woke up from surgery in pain and, at my request, a nurse slammed me in the hand with fentanyl.

Being cut into is a form of trauma, the impact of which depends on individual context. We may consent to this trauma for pleasure or any higher purpose. It is also a release. The cut that enabled the removal of a poisoned part of me in 2018 now feels like a freeing. The burden of a life in an assumed female form, whose inauthenticity had been building in me like a tidal wave, finally began to drain away.

So why did I get cancer? Ten months before the diagnosis, I had started taking combined MHT (menopause hormone therapy). Perhaps these supplemental hormones were responsible? Who knows. Perhaps I am genetically a low-hormone alien, and adding more tipped my cells into confusion.

My visits to hospital were often an ordeal of gendering. Having *miss* and *madam* coming at you is like nails down a blackboard. I went to a patients' meeting where the nurse, otherwise lovely, called us *ladies* every twenty seconds or so. I know this is not simple. Many cis women who have had breast cancer and mastectomies feel they have lost their womanhood, and repeated gendering may be affirming to them. Perhaps it is not, then, a coincidence that *ladies ladies ladies* also echoes throughout the menopause world.

But for me the incongruence of this gendering hit increasingly hard. It invoked in me a kind of misophonia on top of dysphoria. The healthcare industry – and hospitality also – is especially bad for this. Why must people keep informing us of their assumptions?

Ten days after my surgery I went to the clinic to be checked over and be told the successful outcome of the procedure. The consultant noted humorously that my armpit hair, which I had grown out, did not match my head hair. I was fifty-two.

Menopause sits at the intersection of misogyny and ageism. In Western culture, it is traditionally seen as a symbol of redundant femaleness and decrepitude, along with other forms of infertility in bodies with ovarian-based systems. When I went for radiotherapy, I asked for late-morning appointments, but they kept giving me early ones. (*Big deal*, you might say.) However, my overheating and sleeplessness escalated as I went through fifteen sessions of being zapped in a giant machine that a friend said resembled a 'malicious beluga'. Getting up at 7 a.m. to try to be awake enough to get to the hospital felt like an ordeal. When I finally told the technicians that my menopause symptoms were getting worse, and the consequent lack of sleep was impacting my physical and mental health, they glazed over. I felt like I was asking a special favour by asking to be seen later in the day. The weight of shame from this interaction might have caused me to shut up, but it didn't.

In the year that followed I had pain all around my body and experienced an inner exhaustion that felt soul deep – and unfixable by sleep or silence. A year or so after my diagnosis, I woke up one morning unable to walk in a straight line, as if drunk, and for a couple of weeks afterwards I experienced a kind of aura in my head, a vibration that reminded me that I was still on fragile ground. My life's path felt as if it had slimmed to the width of a tightrope.

A counsellor asked me what had been going on in the twelve months up to the diagnosis. That year, in truth, had sickened me. Around the time of the diagnosis, strange symptoms appeared. I was sent for a brain scan and a bowel scan. My relationships were sliding. Just post #MeToo, someone known to many around me was called out for abuse, resulting in protracted fallout. This happens with heartbreaking regularity in sex-positive communities and causes people to step away in droves. My body was responding to the toxicity around me. Nothing could be relied upon.

I was also, with hindsight, undergoing a refit, and a reclaiming.

CHILDHOOD

If you were a boy, you'd probably be GAY! This, from a friend at primary school, was delivered as the ultimate insult. As a young child I played with toy cars, around which I had a rich fantasy life. I played with dolls too. But truly, I preferred vehicles, animals and planets to facsimiles of people.

I wore trousers most of the time – flares, denim and rainbows – and I had an itchy pink 'princess dress' with sequins on it. I built things in the garden. I read piles of books. I loved sci-fi and ghosts and horror. I wanted to be an astronaut. Aged eleven I was full of inventions, plans, structures, drawings. It's taken decades to find that version of me again.

But *tomboy*? No. I didn't understand sports and I struggled to climb things and be upside down (only more recently learning about sensory processing) and lived with the message that I was physically *other*. Any idea that I might be neurodivergent was literally decades away.

As a young teen my height ensured I could perform adulthood sufficiently to get served in pubs. I became the designated drink buyer, just as I was to become the designated driver in my early twenties. Taking risks for others brought a kind of pseudo-maturity. Looking in the mirror, everything felt wrong.

ADULTHOOD

I noted from a young age that people's attention is drawn by several indicators: height, thinness and long hair. For a time, I had all three. Markers in place, I went through the world. My desires, however, did not map onto what was expected of me.

To be read as *female* is to be judged constantly for your appearance. It is hard to be impervious to this. As time passes, and you divert further away from the ideal human module, the age panic some cis-het women experience is hardly surprising. (Aged eighteen, I thought some of my friends' mothers, cis women then in their forties and fifties, were going mad, and I had no idea why.) I will not shame anyone for this, although it does make me weary of patriarchy and the terrible sex and relationships education we receive, and still do.

In my late teens I went from Laura Ashley skirts to a rubber corset, leather trousers and boots. I took pride in certain attributes of my body – my chest – and showed them off. 'They're very big, aren't they!' shouted a friend's mother. Did this make me a woman? Or was this display also a trauma fawn response?* A feminine appearance is also a negotiation. Having breasts felt like a calling card. They drew attention both to me and away from the rest of me at the same time. Double win – I could perform being noticed while hiding!

Much of the time, however, my performance was clearly suboptimal. This recursive reflection sounds like the overthinking that all feminine and assumed-to-be-female people are supposed to suffer from. I look back with some sadness at how, in my younger life, I had fallen into compulsory heterosexuality, and the time I lost to it. Understanding of autistic masking was, again, decades away.

The expectations and disappointments placed on me came in endless flurries. Stories were told on my body. In my mid-twenties I was told I was both too fat and too thin by two different men within the same year. All I remember was navigating endless confusion about what I was supposed to be, and feeling like I was always running behind. I dreamed of living without a physical body at all.

Why did I collude in this for so long? I think that 'woman' was the easiest and nearest person to be. After all, I had the hardware in place. Alien software running on F hardware?

Actually, my software did not work especially well on this hardware. For example, how do you play that game where you pretend to be angry when you're not (to control someone), but hide your genuine anger at other times (to play the game of pretending you're OK with everything to stay safe while you plot)? How do you perform so much just to please others, whether you are feeling it or not? I missed this memo.

---

* A fawn response is when someone attempts to rectify a situation by appeasing the source of the threat and avoiding any further conflict.

I did try, but all those theatrical facial expressions were so, so tiring.

PERIMENOPAUSE

With hindsight, having no information at the time, my perimenopause started in my late thirties and my body did things I did not expect it to do. I had no idea why I was having both terrible mood swings and, simultaneously, a reboot of desire. I started to lose my previously perfect sense of left and right and spent years trying fruitlessly to get help. Up to and after menopause itself, this changing body state made me itch and hurt, and kept me awake with panic, not knowing whether I was too hot or too cold.

Is this how snakes feel when they are about to shed a skin?

It's easy to speak about alienation as an ageing, feminine-presenting person. For the first half of your life you are used to being stared at and hassled, and then it all stops. It's a relief like a kind of secrecy cloak. Everyone has a different experience of it. And now you are pattern-matching and realising the burden of others' expectations that you have been carrying for years.

My perimenopause years were an explosion of joyful self-exploration and validation. But, even then, at any number of play parties, filling my dance card – lots of cleavage and fishnets and boots – even then I wondered what to call myself. Sometimes people would come up to me and admire my chest, which I absolutely enjoyed, while wondering if I had ever been sure what I was.

Perimenopause dragged me from post-sobriety non-sexual self-sheltering into fiery glory. My desires demanded to be free and be seen. I look back on those years mostly with fondness and delight. The clubs, the parties, the workshops, the sweat and the tears. The crying on yoga mats, the laughing sadism, the whip nerdery.

The fire burns brightest when it's about to die down?

POSTMENOPAUSE

'I am loving this Tintin meets Jean Paul Gaultier with a twist of go-go muscle-cub look!' A friend's comment about my grey number-one cut delighted me. Post-cancer I took myself on a two-year hair journey. It was a kind of art project. My hair got shorter with each cut, which I documented on my phone. At the start of the pandemic I rushed to the barber's before lockdown as if a tidal wave was coming.

When wearing a face mask I am often taken for a cis man: I am double-taked in women's toilets and, if a cis woman is trying to get my attention, I have noticed a rising, anxious aggression in tone. Men sometimes take me for one of them, and it's all *boss* and *mate*.

I wear more *men* shirts than *women* shirts. I went from sports bras to compression tops, making clothes that did up with buttons suddenly wearable. I went from owning two shirts to twelve in a year. I don't hugely love the phrase 'nonbinary' – defining someone by what they are not – and I find 'enby'*

---

*A shorthand term meaning 'nonbinary'.

infantilising. But here we are, needing some form of language in order to find each other and show ourselves to the world.

And everyone has their own definition of nonbinary. I have always loved pink, for example, and flowers, but I am also aware that some find this a little suspect. Opportunities for self-gaslighting are legion. The world encourages us to doubt ourselves. I repeat to myself the words: *I don't owe anyone androgyny.*

At the time of writing, my testosterone levels, which tend to lower in menopause along with oestrogen and progesterone (and by the way these hormones are present in *all* bodies), are about as low as they can be for me to remain upright. This feels hard to write and painful. I am not supposed to take *any* hormones, including T, because the cancer was oestrogen-receptor positive and the body can convert testosterone to oestrogen. This frustrates and saddens me daily.

I specifically grieve the postmenopausal loss of muscle mass. I lift weights twice a week when I can, but I could go five times and eat nothing but steamed fish and broccoli and progress would still feel tectonic. However, postmenopause, the gym has been a lifeline for me, and I was overjoyed when I could finally deadlift my own body weight.

Our media, both cis-het and queer, celebrates the colourful, the in-your-face, the extrovert. It similarly celebrates the slim, toned, inverted-triangle body – in all genders. I celebrate all these bodies, while simultaneously looking in.

So what do I do with these 36FFs? I don't hate them, not even close. They can help me project the illusion of a bigger chest. (The paradoxes of dysmorphia!) If I had breast cancer again and needed a mastectomy, I would ask for both to be removed. This, from others' reports, may involve a prolonged dance with gatekeepers.

Menopause has stripped me back and set me free, even while the ageing process is extracting time from me. The experience has been like flying away and looking back at a woman-shaped runway. One of the rewards of this phase of life is that your bullshit detector gets stronger and stronger. Some scenes that I had passed through – and some friendships – just looked like ignorance of power dynamics and poor boundaries.

The menopause world can be positive and generative, but also challenging: the battle of the concave yoga stomachs; the hawking of supplements; the juxtaposition of cis-het wellness culture with queer and trans exhaustion. And of course, the endless gendering of resources and the frequent lack of will to fix this from on high. I experience an increasing divergence from some of my age peers, but a congruent core remains.

Does my story mean that I was, or wasn't, 'born this way'? In some circles there is still an adherence to the idea that if you didn't know your exact, lifelong gender (and sexuality) when you were five years old, you are either faking or delusional or trying to be trendy. (See also neurodivergence.) Others might call this 'born this way or the highway' attitude an aspect of chrononormativity. I welcome the idea that queer lives do not follow the same linear pathways as cis-het ones. (Google 'queer time' or 'queer temporality' and you will end up in theory heaven.)

Do we need to hear other people's stories before we can validate ourselves? I absolutely experience generation envy at times. What if the internet had existed when I was five, twelve or fifteen? Could I have found some kind of mirror?

The cancer was caught early, and at the time of writing has still not recurred. I am a bit dented around the scar, but it feels like a battle trophy. I feel stripped down, as if I had pushed the factory reset button.

Relax, un-perform and *breathe*.

Tania Glyde (they/them) is a London-based psychotherapist and author, specialising in working with gender, sex and relationship diverse (GSRD) clients (londoncentralcounselling.com). They have researched the experiences of LGBTQIA+ menopausal clients in healthcare and are currently working to promote greater understanding of the LGBTQIA+ experience of menopause (queermenopause.com). In 2021 they gave evidence on this subject to the UK House of Commons Women & Equalities Committee. They started the London Gender, Sex and Relationship Therapy Practice (londonsexrelationshiptherapy.com) in 2014 with a group of colleagues. In 2017 they trained as a somatic sexologist. Although their private psychotherapy practice is talk-only, they have found that the opportunity to learn in a somatic (body-based) environment has been invaluable when working with clients. Tania is a published author and has written for the *Lancet* and *Lancet Psychiatry*. In their spare time they enjoy art and weightlifting.

MENOPAUSE HAS STRIPPED ME BACK + SET ME FREE

The Curse of Puberty

Jenn Salib Huber

It's hard to smash the patriarchy on an empty stomach.
Christy Harrison, *Anti-Diet*[1]

Upon crossing the threshold of puberty, boys are celebrated for 'getting so big' and their healthy appetites are kept well fed. A girl, however, will understand the subtext when she's told that she's 'big for her age'. Translation? She's taking up too much space and should keep her growth in check by making herself smaller. She is starting to become too much, and the world doesn't want that from her.

You might be familiar with 'the curse' as a reference to monthly menstrual cycles. Stories referring to the curse of menstruation appear in cultures around the world. 'Eve's curse' – referring, of course, to God's punishment of Eve for enticing Adam to eat the forbidden fruit – is a coming-of-age milestone that everyone blessed with a uterus will experience.

Far be it from me to discount or dismiss the inconvenience of a monthly bleed, the expenses incurred for menstrual 'hygiene' products, or the pain suffered by many women, including me, on a monthly basis. That's not the only curse gifted to us upon crossing the threshold of this reproductive milestone, as the real curse of puberty is the indoctrination into diet culture and the patriarchal concept of the thin ideal that is woven into the fabric of our existence and society. Unlike the burden of periods, this curse doesn't disappear with menopause.

With puberty and the change to our bodies, we become acutely aware of our physical body and how it appears to others. Suddenly we are no longer able to hide behind the anonymity of childhood. We become visible to the world in a way that is unfamiliar, even if not unexpected. Long before we sprout breast buds, we are bombarded with messages about what the 'perfect' body looks like. We're shown images of thin, toned women plastered all over billboards, magazines and social media. Most, if not all, of the dolls on toy shelves share the same idealised hourglass shape. We hear friends and family members talking about dieting and weight loss as if they are keys to happiness and success, and therefore worthy of repeated and endless attempts to succeed. We take note when the discussions around family dinners involve commentary on the shape and size of others' bodies, and worry when comparisons are made to the family members we most resemble.

Thanks to this cultural and social programming, we internalise these messages. We see our bodies as flawed and in need of constant improvement, no matter how exhausting it is to be consumed with thoughts about what our bodies look like to others, or the reflection in our bathroom mirror. We compare and judge our body to those around us. We begin to see food as the enemy and obsess over calories, macros and portion sizes. We become experts at disguising our hunger and denying ourselves the pleasure of food in order to fit into the narrow confines of the thin ideal. No one has yet told us that we can't hate ourselves into a body that we love.

Even more insidious is that dieting is framed as virtuous, normalised even, and applauded under the veil of 'healthy eating'. We are told that we are simply taking care of ourselves, that we are being healthy and responsible by obsessively watching what we eat. We are encouraged to view our bodies as projects that we can (and should) constantly try to improve upon, rather than as living, breathing beings that deserve to live peacefully just as we are. Even overtly disordered behaviours like skipping meals and over-exercising aren't a problem unless we become 'too thin'. And it's all in an attempt to conform to the impossible standards that have been set for us to remain attractive to the male gaze, but also serves to keep us subdued and distracted. As Naomi Wolf writes in *The Beauty Myth*: 'Dieting is the most potent political sedative in women's history; a quietly mad population is a tractable one.'

I started my period just before my tenth birthday, positioning me at the front of my peer group. Accordingly, I was the first to become acutely aware of the hierarchy of bodies in the playground, the importance of clothing size and weight as symbols of acceptance and belonging, and the shame of growing out instead of up. By the time I turned twelve, I was the first to feel that I was taking up too much space. Baggy clothes and slouched shoulders became the norm as I attempted to hide the shame I felt in, and about, my body.

My first diet would be fuelled by a moment of self-loathing brought on by a bathing suit not fitting the way I expected it to. My newly soft and rounder body felt awkward and unfamiliar, and I vividly remember the reflection in the mirror feeling alien to what had (and hadn't) been there just months before. The elastic waistband of the bottoms pinched at my now curvy hips, and the top looked far too much like a bra to feel safe and comfortable in my body. If only I'd been told that my body needed to change, and that the increase in body fat was programmed into my DNA. If only I'd been taught that weight was not a behaviour.

Salads led to SlimFast shakes, followed by skipped lunches and Lean Cuisine. By my fifteenth birthday I had become an actual poster child for a local diet centre, my photo gracing the pages of our local paper as a testimonial to their success. I was proof that dieting worked. I had *arrived* and was enjoying existing in a body that was praised and accepted. I enjoyed being admired, and it wasn't just from boys, or friends who had previously been just outside the reach of my social circle. Teachers, friends and even their parents were quick to congratulate me on my success. One pinned my newspaper photo to their fridge for inspiration. The photo remained long after my fifteen minutes of fame had passed, but served as a constant reminder of what was expected of me, and my body.

I was fifteen. Still young enough to have a handful of stuffed animals on my bed, and Barbie dolls still visible at the back of my closet. Yet my brief but powerful experience of living in a smaller body convinced me unequivocally that my weight defined my worth. I could never have imagined how much work it would take to uncouple those beliefs.

I wasn't alone, either. Girls all around me were going through the same thing, struggling to fit in and be accepted in a world that demanded perfection. We were all trying to navigate a system that was rigged against us, constantly bombarding us with messages that we were not good enough as we were. We *could* always be better, if we tried hard enough. Magazines for tweens and teens offered up food and exercise advice to flatten our stomachs and ways to get the 'perfect' back-to-school hair, with no attempt to hide that getting boys' attention was the ultimate goal. It has been reported that 53 per cent of thirteen-year-old American girls are unhappy with their bodies. This grows to 78 per cent by the time girls reach 17.[2] Other studies have found that 46 per cent of nine- to eleven-year-olds are sometimes or very often on diets, as are 82 per cent of their families.[3] If only my indoctrination into diet culture was the exception, not the rule.

By the time I was eighteen, and getting ready to leave for university, I had graduated from successful dieter to chronic dieter. It wouldn't occur to me that anything I was doing was harmful or even abnormal until many years later. I chose to study nutrition, convinced that becoming a dietitian would ensure my future success as a dieter. The cure for my lack of thinness was, I believed, more knowledge. Through my studies, the secret to easy, sustainable weight loss would be revealed to me, or so I thought. The problem was that I was unknowingly surrounded by people (mostly women) who also felt broken and were in need of fixing. One-third of dietetic students are motivated to enter the field by personal experiences (self or friends) with weight or eating disorders.[4] Some do graduate as 'normal eaters' with a healthy relationship with food and a strong distrust of the multibillion-dollar diet industry. Many others, like I did, hide disordered eating under the umbrellas of health and wellness culture, because when diet culture fails us, wellness culture is quick to jump in and save us.

The true cost of staying in diet culture in pursuit of the thin ideal would not become evident until after my children were born. When the surgeon who performed my caesarean section came to check on me in the hospital, he reassured me with a wink that my scar would not be visible if I wanted to wear a bikini. Articles about how to 'get your body back' after having a baby were found in every parenting magazine, including the ones in my doctor's office. It was impossible to escape the message that remaining attractive was still very much expected of me. Suddenly I became aware that these concepts were deeply rooted in patriarchy, in a subversive attempt to control and dominate women's bodies in order to maintain power and control over them. I was able to see that the beauty standards imposed upon me were not based on objective reality but, rather, on a long history of misogyny, racism and oppression.

Despite being marketed under the guise of health, diet culture is not about health or wellbeing. It's about profit and control. The diet industry is worth billions of dollars and thrives on making women feel inadequate and insecure about their bodies. It sells us false promises of happiness and success that, in reality, only lead to more shame and self-hatred when nothing works as we hoped. It's often not until we've invested over half of our lives that we see that we haven't failed at dieting. Dieting has failed us.

Pursuing a body shape that only represents 5 per cent of the diversity of human bodies is not without risk. Studies show that the constant pressure to conform to the thin ideal leads not only to eating disorders, disordered eating and body dysmorphia, but depression, anxiety and even hormonal imbalances, all of which can have long-term effects on our overall health and wellbeing.

The patriarchy is deeply invested in maintaining the thin ideal as a means of keeping women in a state of perpetual insecurity and self-doubt. Who has time to challenge the status quo or demand equal rights and opportunities when we're preoccupied with our appearance? We are more likely to be compliant and docile, willing to conform to the expectations of others rather than asserting our own needs and desires. This is the real curse of puberty. At a time of great change and transition – a time when we are most vulnerable to the messages and expectations of the culture around us – we need others to lift us up. Instead, they let us down with their opinions and judgements.

Like puberty, menopause is another reproductive milestone in a woman's life that is greeted with mixed emotions. For some (including me) it's a welcome end to decades of menstrual pain and discomfort. For others it's greeted with a bittersweet mix of gratitude and grief. Gratitude for the end of decades of menstrual hassle: pain, discomfort and expense. Grief for the loss of our youth, made all the more obvious as our bodies change once again. With our hormones shifting, the much maligned 'meno-belly' often emerges. Once again our body image and self-esteem suffer because of the unrealistic expectation set by a culture obsessed with thinness. Is it really so hard to accept that it's normal for human bodies to change?

Menopause has become a commodity, and the lucrative dieting industry has wasted no time in creating solutions to our midlife body changes. With no effort at all, it's easy to find diets, pills, books and workouts promising to cure 'meno-belly'. Of course, there is no magic cure to be found as, just like changes in puberty, this change is preprogrammed into our DNA.

Like so many other aspects of midlife, much of what comes with the menopause is unexpected, if not unwelcome. The rollercoaster of hormone changes alters what our body looks like, so that our physical self feels like a shape-shifting interloper caught on an alien planet. And it comes with decades of programming telling us we need to fight it. Harder. And NOW. Most of us do, at least for a while.

As we wind our way down hormonally in our forties or fifties, we cross over with a younger version of ourselves, long lost to diet culture. If we're listening, we might hear the whisper of a voice inviting us to surrender in the decades-long battle with our body. We can finally end the war that has distracted us from *living* in the body we have.

Even if we call a truce, the sense of loss is somewhat inevitable. As we grieve the thin ideal and move through the stages of grief, anger awakens at the realisation that the battle has been a war with ourselves. The real enemy has tricked us into believing that our bodies were the problem. We've devoted years of our lives to fixing something that was never broken, and now bear the scars of the battles we've fought.

Midlife and menopause can make us more discerning of who, and what, is deserving of our time and energy. No becomes easier to say than yes, especially if saying yes comes at a cost we're no longer willing to pay. It was during my perimenopausal years that I realised I was no longer willing to pay the price to continue trying to hate myself into a body I could love. I was no longer willing to suffer to meet the expectations of others. I would no longer keep trying to make myself smaller. The curse I'd carried for nearly thirty years had been lifted.

Many parts of my personal and professional journey to food and body freedom had to be walked alone. I am grateful that I crossed paths with intuitive eating relatively early on, providing me with the framework to redefine my relationship with food. Like so many of the women I now work with, I didn't know how to eat if I wasn't chasing a number on the scale. Intuitive eating introduced me to gentle nutrition, and to trust that my body could lead me to foods that I wanted and needed.

In menopause, food matters. How we nourish ourselves in this stage of life matters. Nutrition can have a big impact on not only how we feel, but also how we age. Independence, mobility and strength require fuel. Our brain, heart and bones are adapting to the loss of oestrogen and need us to support them in sustainable yet flexible ways. Diets are neither sustainable nor flexible, which is why I've made it my mission to help women manage menopause without diets and food rules.

Breaking the curse for ourselves is only part of what we must do. Saving our daughters from the curse weakens the shackles of the patriarchy that has wanted to keep us small. Menopause is an opportunity to lift the curse. It is our time to live *in* our bodies and embody the power we possess.

> At her first bleeding a woman meets her power.
> During her bleeding years she practices it.
> At menopause she becomes it.
>
> Traditional Native American saying

Dr Jenn Salib Huber (she/her) is a Canadian Registered Dietitian, naturopathic doctor and certified intuitive eating counselor, and she's on a mission to help women thrive in midlife. She helps women navigate the physical and emotional changes that happen in perimenopause and menopause, including their search for food freedom and body confidence. Working from a 'health at every size' approach, she teaches women to become intuitive eaters and build body confidence at any stage of midlife.

SHE IS STARTING TO BECOME **TOO MUCH**

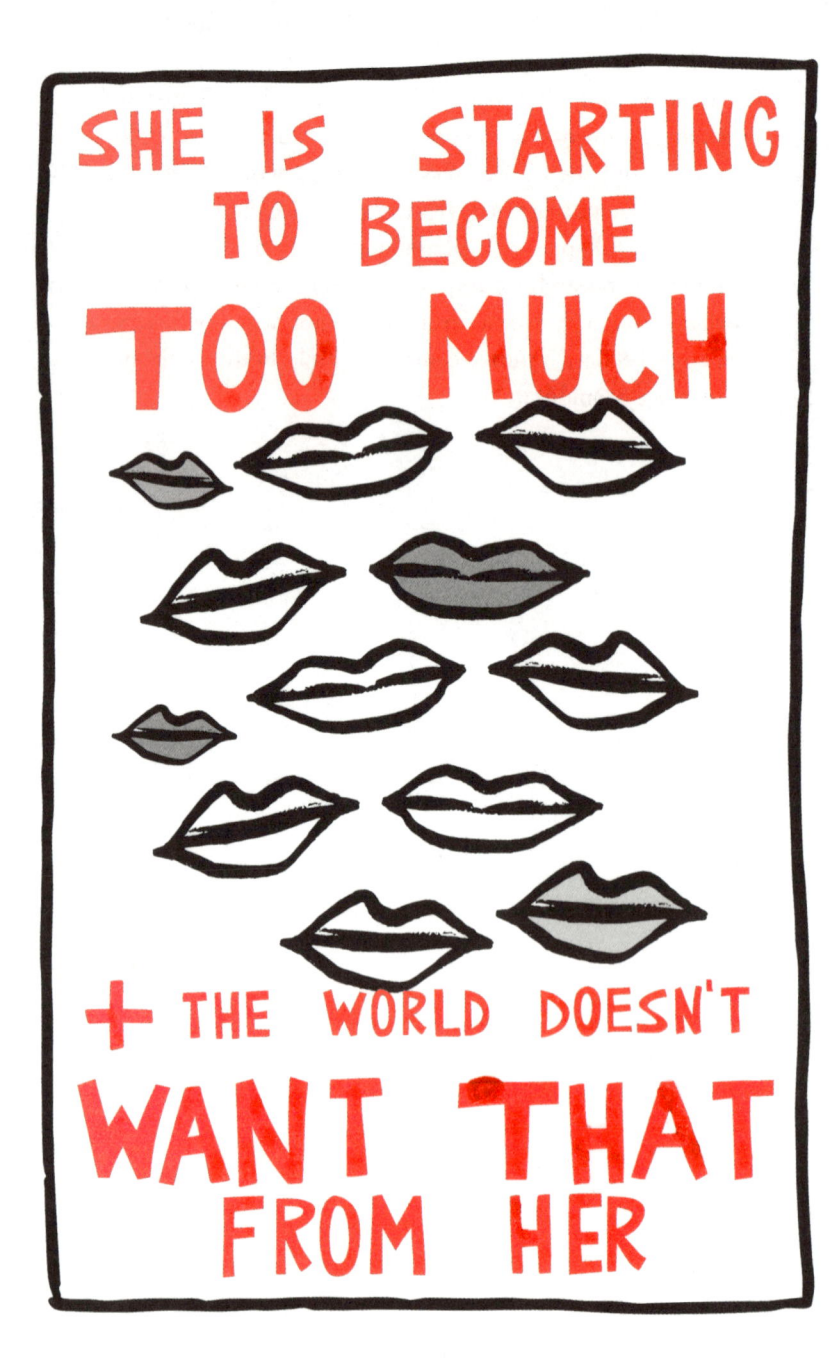

+ THE WORLD DOESN'T **WANT THAT FROM HER**

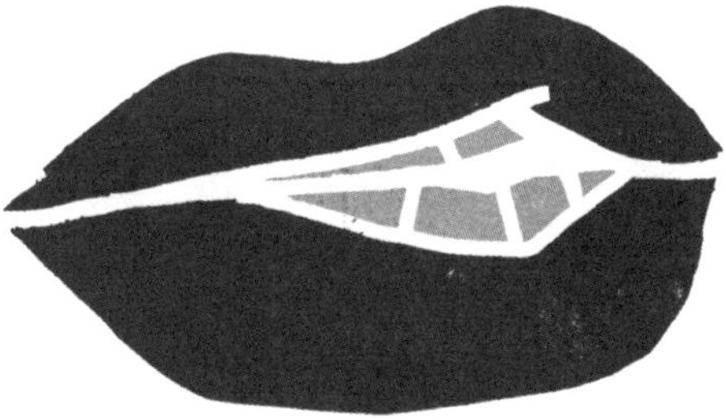

I BECAME BOTH **FEARLESS** + **FANCIFUL**

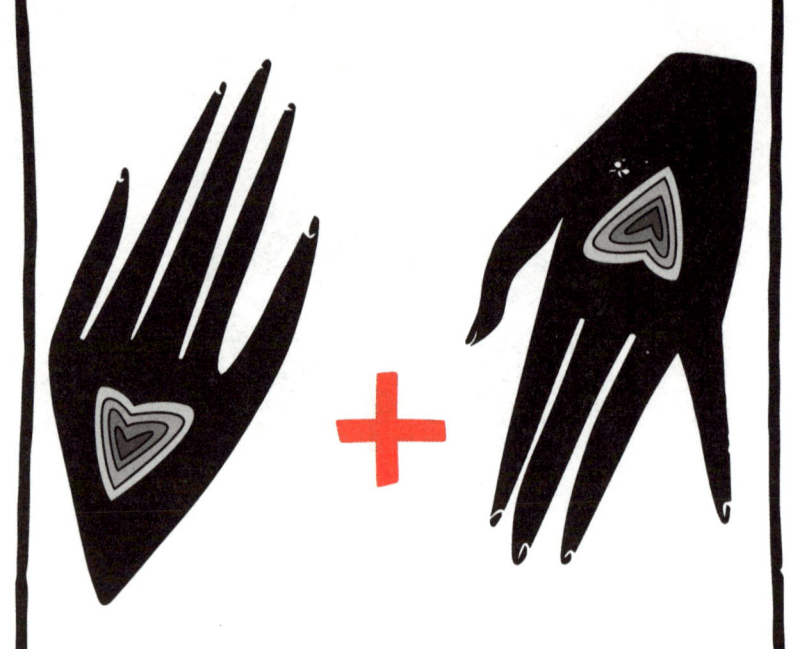

Don't Bring a Flashlight to the Brain Fog

Sonora Jha

Menopause changes my sweet smile into a smirk, and 'I love that for me,' as the kids say.

Don't get me wrong. I am not trying to put a positive spin on menopause or anything. It's been brutal, dear reader. There's nothing pretty about it. Indeed, I watch as it takes all conventional notions of prettiness and sucks the moisture out of it, just as the word 'dewy' becomes all the rage in the beauty industry.

This is fine, I tell myself, like the meme of the dog in the fire, and yet there's nothing memetic about the literal sense of fire I feel under my breezy cotton tee in winter, just like there is nothing memetic (as in a well-propagated cultural idea) about menopause, of which we know shit. This is fine, I tell myself, because who cares about dewy prettiness when I have a brain and a book contract?

But I digress. And I digress because, darlings, what I am trying to say is that I have brain fog, one of the least talked-about symptoms of menopause, and it gives me permission to mix my metaphors to tell you that I am in the thick of it.

But as I was saying, the smirk is a thing of beauty. My smile no longer hints at sweetness or surrender; it is sardonic and self-satisfied, and it represents the journey I am going to tell you about, from the beginnings of the brain fog in perimenopause to the clarity offered by my recent postmenopausal state.

It began with the return of 'the daydreaming'. As a child, I would spend hours staring into space, daydreaming about nothing in particular. This led to my teachers and other adults and children around me declaring me 'slow', 'stupid' and 'a failure'. My teacher in the first standard (first grade) declared me 'weak at mathematics', and the condemnation stuck (in India, if you were weak in mathematics, you sorry thing, you would die poor and lonely). But the thing about failure is that it frees you up from other people's expectations, and mine freed me up for daydreaming, which lasted from age six to around nineteen. Three decades later, I found myself daydreaming again.

Lots of staring into space as the clock ticked by. Hours and hours of nothing but looking out on the lake outside my Seattle condo as the light changed on the water. While in my girlhood this daydreaming felt like some sort of freedom, it struck terror in my heart now. This time around it was understood to be brain fog, the perimenopausal symptom few people know of and fewer people take seriously.

My entire life is built around my brain. Letting it fog up could be devastating to my career as a professor, a researcher, a writer with contracts to write two books in my peak menopausal years. Other symptoms of menopause were physical and therefore seemed more or less manageable with some insight and planning. For instance, I ordered a tower fan to stand two feet from my bed and carefully programmed its smart settings to sync up with my night sweats. I put some serious money down for a Peloton for the extra-extra pounds that I predicted would lovingly cling to me because my menopause coincided with the stillness of a pandemic. I hung on for dear life to my therapist for the rising anxiety and the looming possibility of depression. I scheduled time with friends for 'a sense of being needed'.

But I also signed those book contracts for 'a sense of purpose', and now here I was, grinning slack-jawed for hours at the way my dog nodded off to sleep by the fireplace or the way the squirrel in the tree defied gravity, or have you ever noticed how . . .

Words started to disappear from my head. In conversations or meetings, I started to replace the lost words with 'that thing', or 'thingy', or the 'you know what I'm referring to', or the 'what's it called'. I lost my ability to focus, especially on the written word. Everything I have to my name is built on the written word. I trade in the written word. The Hindu goddess I worship is Saraswati, the goddess of, among other things, the written word. My pay cheque arrives in my bank and goes instantly to the bank of my mortgage lender because of my hard work on the written word. And now the written word may as well have been a squirrel's droppings across the page . . . well, maybe, the way I was going, a squirrel's droppings would be something I could stare at for hours. Not so much the written word.

'Have you tried audiobooks?'

I have wanted to scream a horror-movie graveyard scream into the face of anyone who suggests this. Yes, I had tried audiobooks and I'd hated them. But I was willing to try anything to keep my mind now, so I smiled my smirky smile and tried audiobooks again, and this time they were glorious. They helped me stare into space with a story playing in my ear. My mind still wandered into the fog, but a good turn of phrase works magic on 'the change of life'. Thanks to these wondrous things, I hid with quite some success my inability to read words on a page.

I found ways to become a functioning daydreamer.

I showed up on time for my Zoom meetings but forgot if I had showered that day. I could focus enough to make lesson plans for classes to teach but I could no longer depend on my ability to go off the cuff and be the brilliant teacher whose wisdoms were in her head, to pull out like glittering gems in response to dazzling questions. Now all wisdoms were in bullet points to pull out in PowerPoints. I'd stare straight into faces of friends and colleagues, know I loved them, but not know their names. And then there was the morning when I set out to walk my dog in my thin, transparent, pyjama bottoms and only realised it three blocks and a hundred stares later. Where was the invisibility of ageing womanhood when I needed it?

Here's the thing – I had no idea what was happening to me. Yes, I knew I was perimenopausal, but the only symptoms that I had heard of in the patriarchosphere were hot flashes, anger, vaginal dryness and weight gain. Not surprisingly, I had heard of the symptoms that represented the manifestations that would mess with my appearance to others, the experience of me by others or in relationship with others. Yes, hot flashes were personal experiences, but the discussion around them is usually about how to deal with them when they occur in company – who wants to break out in sweat or turn red during a work meeting?

Brain fog, on the other hand, is a slow burn. Yes, the culture makes jokes about women losing their minds, turning dull or forgetful as they age, but if I had heard of it as a symptom of menopause, I would not have been so totally terrified or felt so staggeringly alone. I eventually came around to embracing the daydreaming and claiming for myself this cow-like state as somewhat delectable (if one must, at different points of a woman's life, be described as having bovine qualities such as lactating or being an 'old cow', one may as well also embrace being a 'mad cow'). But the road to making such peace with my 'pause was, well, foggy.

I tried to research my way out of it. I am, after all, an academic, a researcher, a scholar (for whom menopause came, nonetheless). After poring through books and papers that warned me of Alzheimer's disease and dementia, I found myself dwelling on a research paper titled 'Menopause as a stage of female development: psychoanalytic perspective', published by two Russian women academics, E. S. Mordas and A. G. Kuz'micheva, in *Psychologist* in 2021. The authors' research found that how a woman reacts to changes brought about by menopause depends on her individual mental development and sociocultural factors. In general, women tend to deny the bodily changes and the associated affective responses of menopause. Denial is a woman's primary defence and is often expressed by a level of increased activity, career advancement, the belief that you can 'restart' your life. Women try to organise the chaos.

It all tracked for me. Denial, rooted in shame, was the way I was raised to treat my body. The name given to the vulva in my childhood in India was 'shame-shame'. I grew up in urban, English-speaking, middle-class Indian environments. I suspect this, or some version of this, is what vulvas were called in other families, too. The reason I don't know this for sure is that no one referenced vulvas at all, for the reasons implied by the name – they were about shame, twice over. Any time my body demanded attention – in puberty, in pregnancy, in multiple surgeries on my ankles after a car crash and a renewed complication from childhood polio – my mind swooped in to offer a hyperfocus. I toiled over maths at thirteen. I did the best stories of my journalism career at twenty-six in Bangalore, in the months of my pregnancy. I researched and wrote a whole Ph.D. dissertation from my wheelchair after those surgeries.

In the brain fog of menopause, I did meticulous interviews, researched, wrote and edited a memoir and then revised and edited a novel. I met every writing deadline set by my publisher. In other words, I exhausted myself by pushing my brain and ramping up my stress around how it was trying to outsmart me into dullness.

I did similar hijinks with my body. The research, particularly an oft-cited one by Helene Deutsch published in 1984 with the minimalist title 'The menopause', published in *The International Journal of Psychoanalysis*, pointed to a resurgence in libidinal activity, 'a narcissistic need to be desired and loved', a revolt against the casting of the older woman as asexual, undesirable, unattractive.

This, too, tracked for me. Three months into a global pandemic in which we were forbidden to breathe around strangers, I met a man online and invited him in to breathe hard with me as a lover. Never had I ever taken a risk of any kind in my sexual life; in fact, I had always been cast as 'the good girl', and later, between and after my divorces, the 'infrequent dater', with sexual partners I could count on the fingers of one hand. Now, with brain fog, here I was, fogging up the windows as this man and I took road trips across the state of Washington.

Deutsch also spoke of a woman's tendency, in this phase of her life, to experience 'vaginal frustration', and to 'move from reality to fantasy'. Other researchers speak of women wanting to separate from and reassess their relationships. It didn't take me long to reassess my relationship with the pandemic-time lover. I ended it because I was bored and desired to return to the state of solitude I had come to, finally and unexpectedly, enjoy in the months of the pandemic. I was a twice-divorced empty-nester. I wasn't supposed to enjoy isolation; in fact, cultural cues had always been so strong against any settling into a state of single-old-woman bliss that I didn't see it coming to wrap me like a soft, intricately embroidered pashmina shawl.

Which is what brings me to how I eventually reframed, recast and, indeed, relished the brain fog.

In the silence, the solitude and the staring into space, I found a bliss on which I couldn't pin down a description. I took stock of how much storage space I was using up in my brain and what I was storing there. It is commonly thought that we only use 10 per cent of our brains, although scientists dispute that. I was using mine to store dates, memories, trauma, hopes, despair and dreams. My inventory led to a spring cleaning. Was it that my brain was now feeling the rush of empty space as it was finally free of the minutiae that must be stocked in a mother's head? Was a part of it emptied out of a load of years of folders, files and calendars of my kid's schedules of school and extracurriculars and social life, and my own tenure and promotion clock, and a needlessly packed schedule of work and gym and social and romantic partnership and community scheduling that assemble themselves into a woman's life? I mean, the sheer relief of not having to track one's period alone was a whole portal into which thin air could now rush in and float around.

What if I decided to let this fog be as it was, let it float and burn and slow me down and make me forgetful and slow and sleepy?

I wasn't being irresponsible. In fact, I would definitely challenge my brain so it didn't turn to cotton – but instead of feeling frantic and full, and instead of struggling against the brain fog, I'd let it now focus on whatever it fancied. If I can't read, I let reading fall away from my head. I listen to music instead, and I sing the lyrics out loud. I do a daily Wordle. I peer with wonder at the way the viburnum flowers of one tree mingle with the magnolias of another at this one corner on my morning walk with my dog. Indeed, I let myself follow his sniffs and I look at the green of grass as if I am seeing it for the first time. What does my brain want to know about green grass?

I also found a new form of clarity – I found a mind and voice that cut to the chase in work meetings, relationships and creative thinking. I found an eloquence in my rage when I needed to write a feminist essay. I called bullshit on systems of inequity at work. I became both fearless and fanciful in my dating life, which means that I refused to settle. I nurtured my solitude and amplified my laughter in all settings, which is to say I let myself become that woman who laughs too loudly.

I decided I wouldn't bring a flashlight to the brain fog. I took a leap of faith into the fog. I now allow myself to fail a little. I did not meet the deadline for this essay. I asked for an extension, and I savoured the slow storytelling that my brain seems to want of me.

I want to now take conversations of menopausal brain out of the whisper network and shout this from the rooftops – your brain might be telling you to get some rest, dwell on things other than keys and directions and matching socks. It may be inviting you to daydream, to wonder, to wander into the fog and return, smirking with a quiet wisdom.

Sonora Jha, Ph.D. (she/her) is the author of three books, including the novels *The Laughter* (2023), *Foreign* (2013) and the memoir *How to Raise a Feminist Son* (2021). She was a journalist in India and Singapore before moving to the United States. She is a professor of journalism and an associate dean at Seattle University. Her new novel, about a menopausal woman who lines up suitors to perform a feat to win her hand in marriage, is forthcoming in 2025.

I FOUND A BLISS, A NEW CLARITY, AN ELOQUENCE IN MY RAGE

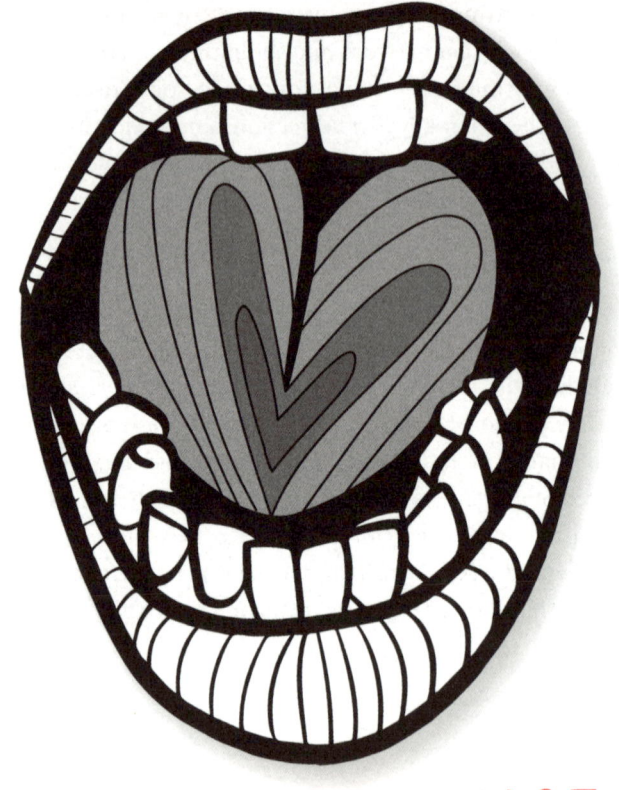

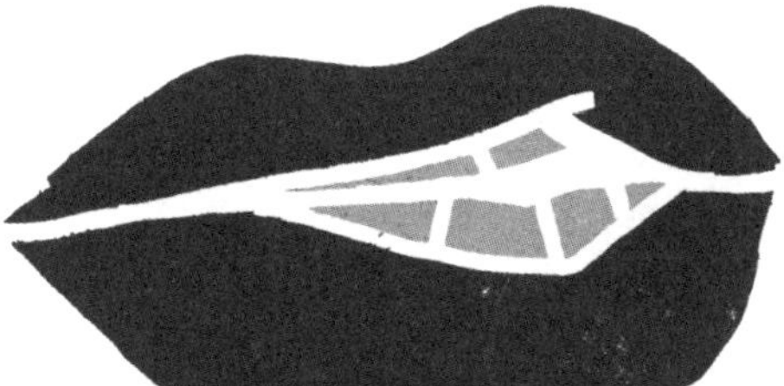

GENDER IS AS MULTITUDINOUS AS WAVES

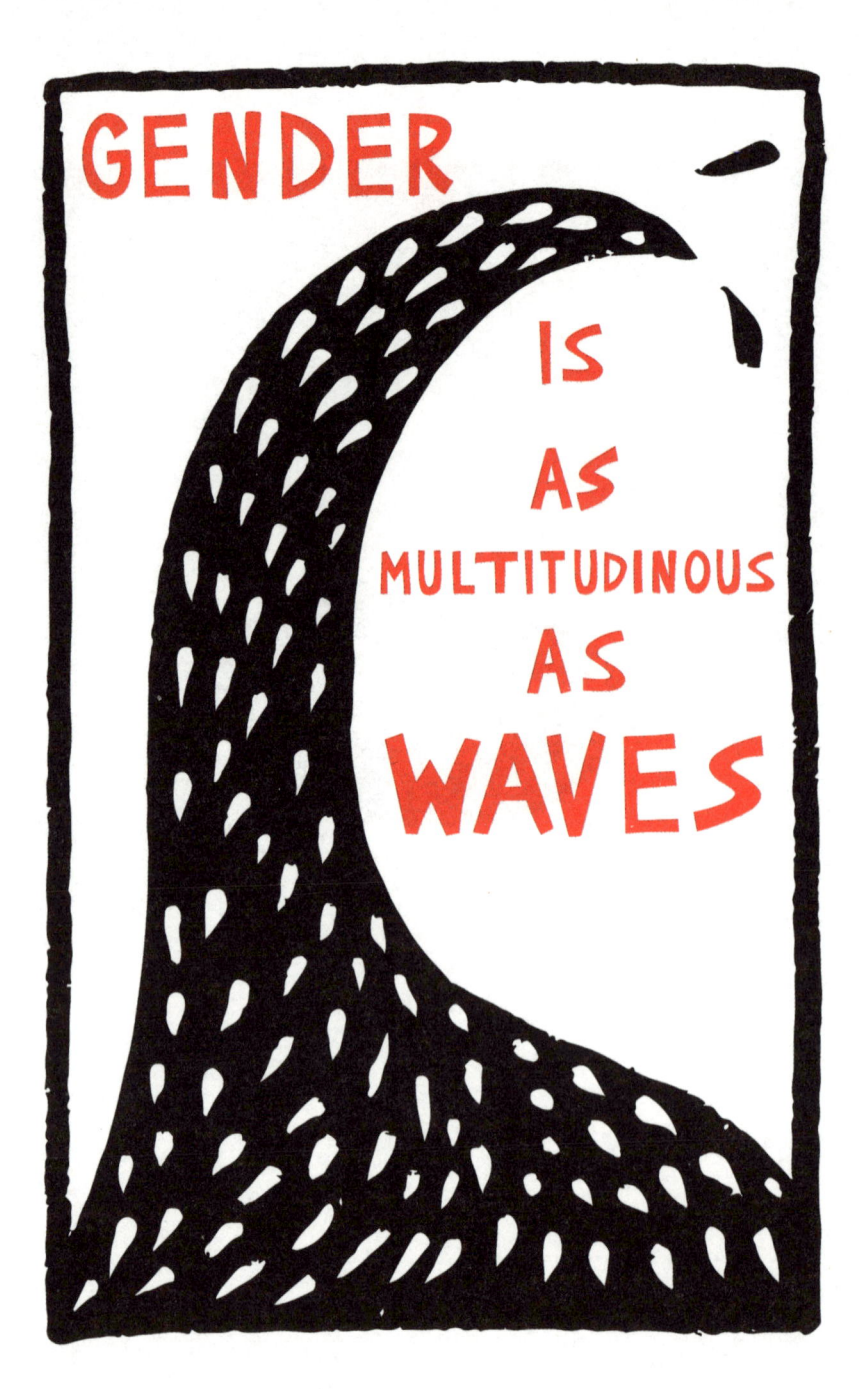

Lost Pages from the Lore of Menses /
كتابات الفائضات في نزهات الحائضات

Mohja Kahf

They ask thee concerning Menses and Women. Say ye: Women and All People with Wombs.

We created you-all from a single Self of no gender or all genders, and it was Beautiful and True. From that One Nafs flowed and differentiated another Self that was Beautiful and True and it, too, had no gender or all genders. From the equal twain flowed and flowered and were differentiated all the many genders.

On the authority of our Mother Hawwa, parent of the brothers Abeel and Habeel and their sisters Sawdaa and Sha3thaa and their khuntha siblings Layl and Nur: A river runs through you. May it keep you tender. Neither a curse nor a pollution, it is your moisture like tears are the moisture of your eyes. Let it pour into a soft chalice inside your Vagina; you may use it to fertilise your tulip bulbs. When it is gone, you may feel a type of way, but each of you may feel a different type of way. And I herald for you an Age of Abundancy, when the river opens its mouth unto the ocean and sweet and salt waters meet each other without losing each their distinct qualities. How doth your body?

On the authority of Hajar wo Mombasa, Mother of the Believers in the Wholesomeness of Women's Bodies, narrated by her niece Tamiqua Jackson, that her great-grandmother, who was a Companion of the Person Who Loved Her Period, Bibi Sidra the Truthteller (MDEH – May the Divine Empower Her), said:

Behold, my period comes. I start feeling melted and sexy a night or two before, and want to be held tenderly and protectively and made love to mightily, and then I want to be covered gently and left to sleep a bonus sleep off the clock, no babies no dishes no phone. And that is how I know it is coming, and it feels like an old friend whose face I love. For behold, I love my period. (She said this latter three times.)

Says the teacher Cho Sonsaeng (MTBBC – May They Be Blessed Continually): Behold, I feel like a truck runneth over my body and I want none, nay none, to touch me; I retreat for Self-care out the Wazoo.

Said Sri Saudari Maryam: Orgasm relieves menstrual cramping. Do not hold her at bay. But if she holds you at bay then do not push against her. Some People with Periods cannot abide to be touched during their periods, while others need to be touched. How doth your Body?

And the people of Ignorance said: Here comes bint khaltek, Um Kulsoum, that time of the month, Aunt Flow, cranberry woman. On the rag. Ya muftra ya mum, ya shakhakhet dum.

And the Truthteller replied instead: Verily and merrily, the moon has been sighted from the hilltop; let the festivities begin! I'm driving my red convertible. Queen Zumurrud unwinds her red turban. Roll out the red carpet.

And the seventh layer of Commentators added: Listen. This is what it sounds like to hear from your ancestors words that love Women and all People with Wombs. Words that do not make Women curl up and die inside.

But Hajar wo Mombasa (MSBGP – May She Be Given Pleasure) said, regarding both narratives: Just call it what it is, yoh. Enough with silly code words.

They ask thee concerning Menarche. Say, Menarche is a time of threshold. Prepare, prepare. Let the Young One know in the years before. For verily, the hormones cometh. My Little One, you're becoming a woman now (but hey, you're still a Little One in other ways, for many years, and it is still our job to generate for you safety and nurturance). How doth your body fare? You may not find clothes that fit – retailers don't listen to real girls' bodies and make clothes for this age, neither a little girl any more nor yet a woman fully. Capitalism says wear this, wear that – seek guidance, but you decide. Religions say wear this, wear that – seek guidance, but you decide. Elderwomen in Damascus once cooked seven-grain pudding and served it in the neighbourhood to celebrate with sweetness the child's first period, a trace from ancient goddess rites honouring our fertility (instead of fearing it).

Little One, if your body seems wrongly gendered to you, like a heavy glove over your inner truth, know you are Loved by the Ineffable Divine. And Benign Elders will help you in your Path. And may your Inner Being shine.

And Sri Saudari Maryam the Truth-Bearer noted interlinearly: If these words seem strange to you, it is because you have become accustomed not to honour and love all possible genders.

They ask thee concerning gender; say, Ye Gender is multitudinous as ocean waves. Each with distinct shape and qualities, crest and foam, yet each as One with the Whole Ocean.

Mention in the matter the khuntha, indeterminate and many-formed, floating through our Lore. Behold, in Arabic orthography the word's end is rounded full-bellied feminine, yet the word takes a male gender, thus toggling indeterminacy throughout the sentence. Part of our language and our heritage, khuntha always had a space to Pray that was neither with the men nor with the Women. They were always There.

Embrace ye Perplexity, sayeth Ibnat al-Arabi.

And mention the ghulamiya, bearing a boyish name-kernel and a hinting face, yet a feminine-knotted rear-ending and trace. Playful is her moustache. Or his moustache, or theirs? Slim as it is, zir moustache contains multitudinous layers. Floats the ghulamiya through Abbasid corridors, yet different from the khuntha, a different blending.

Remember ye the mukhannathoon of Medina were men in body yet Women in kohl and paint, and spoke with each other using the feminine grammatical forms, yet lay not with each other, or some may have lain but others not; ye may know them Knot by their outward forms. Welcomed in the home of the Prophet, the differently gendered have always been There in our history.

Behold, there are many others whose secrets ye shall not know, illegible they in the sublunary world.

Verily the Lasting into which the soul upon annihilation dissolves hath no gender but is the Utter Absence of gender in all its multiplicity and specificity, in superlunary realms Beyond the Lote Tree of the Ultimate. Beyond Binary, beyond boundary. Ponder that, ye that would ponder.

Says Ibnat al-Labbanah: I am luminous and planetary. Not inscribed in my body is my truth.

And Ibn Nafsihi narrates in *The Necklace of Rarest Gemstones* in the Black Opal Chapter that Hasan al-Basri once saw a person levitating over the Tigris River near the Street of the Apothecaries, and recognised Zir and knew Zhe was the valiant khuntha Mutawwaj and asked, O Mutawwaj, will ye [and al-Basri, speaking Arabic, used the dual grammatical form] come to port on the Kharkh side or the Rusafa side? And Mutawwaj said: By the Ineffable who gives me the power to levitate over sweet waters and salt waters, I shall cross fully neither to one riverbank nor the other. Twilight, dusk and Estuaries know me.

And this has been erased from the Lore by redactors of an Age That Could Not Puzzle its meaning, so they tore the page from the book or reddened the lines with blotches of red ink.

And still the tedious authorities of the Days of Rejection said: Here is a list of things you are forbidden to do during menses. Pray. Fast. Make love. Make tawaf. Enter a mosque.

But She who Bore Truth during the Days of Rejection (MGSHQ – May God Strengthen Her Questioning) questioned: Why is The God You Think Of a 'he' when The Divine is Ineffable? The God You Think Of leaves me in despair. The Ineffable hath said: I Am as my worshipper thinks I Am. So I do not think of the Ineffable as you think. They are Beyond.

And the Divine says: My Womb-mercy prevails over my wrath. And Maryam, Mother of Essa, prayed to al-Rahman.

And, Full of Grace, the Mothers of Moses, Jesus and Muhammad said in unison: Rahma comes from Rahm. For the Divine is UnBodily and Unspeakable in human grammar. Pray, then, if you are among the Prayers, without gendering the Divine. Or if ye must gender, alternate. And grow in Divine Bewilderment.

And God sayeth 'We'. And They have sometimes used 'he' as a grammatical placeholder. But Those Who Rejected People with Wombs cried: Though we admit with our lips that God is neither He nor She, in our hearts we limit God to 'he'. And his Jalal overrules his Jamal, with us.

And the people of the Days of Rejection enquired of the Bleeding Womb-bearer: Are you fasting, or aren't you fasting? Are you praying, or aren't you praying? Are you pure, or are you impure? Are you polluted on Mount Arafat? (Even this they dare say.) Is your Hajj viable? (Imagine, this they dare say!) And they just would not stop. And their binary thinking led them to Hell of Their Own Making.

Our Mother Hawwa (MHMBB) said: No descendant of ours shall call themselves impure or polluted by way of bodily functions. No human being is impure in that way, for pollution is what comes to the soul from deliberately causing great suffering, as does a tyrant. No living creature is impure. All living creatures have souls. Also, all animals are Muslim and have communities in Paradise. [Note of the Fourth Redactor: The Malikis still hold to this Clean Souls Doctrine, and hold with paradise for dogs and cats and horses and octopuses and other creatures.] Therefore do not insult your own Soul by calling anybody impure. [And it is not clear if the latter is part of what was narrated or part of the Commentary of later layers of Commentators.]

Lost Pages from the Lore of Menses | 85

And via Pari-khan the Pearl Diver who heard it from her great-aunt Nzinga Liu who heard it from the Companion Fatima Swift Swimmer, our Mother Hawwa added: Honey, you can too swim during your period. Enjoy the pool and the beach! But the Haters of People with Wombs tried to fasten all the waters of the earth, to keep the Waters for themselves only. Lo, Water and Sun and Wind and Earth are the greatest hujjahs and allies to Women and all People with wombs. Have we not made the Water, Sun and Wind caress you when you are melancholy, and for you to caress the Earth with your planting hands brings you joy?

And Our Mother Hawwa (MHMBB) added: You may hear ugly stories about me but do not believe them. I, your Ancestor Who Loves You, was never cursed by the Ineffable Divine; I was blessed. Verily, your period is one of the Signs of Rahmana, so learn to read the Divine markings in your underknickers.

So the People with Wombs in Medina used to send Aisha pieces of cloth from between their thighs to ask her learned opinion. How shall we read the yellow markings? How the brown spots? For Aisha was a lore-learned woman. And they used to light lanterns in the night to check their innermost undergarments.

And Cho Sonsaeng (MTBBC) commented here: Contemplation of this can lead to elevated spiritual states.

Added the Eleventh Redactor: Even still, some will raise their hands and ask: Teacher, can I recite Quran when I am menstruating? Can I pick it up if I am dusting the shelf? Can I recite a whole sura or part of a sura? Can I recite kul a'uthu bi rab al-nas if I am in fear? And the Sonsaeng (MTBBC) said: Of course you can, and these are questions of those living in the Set of Rules made by men who do not honour Women, Femmes and People with Wombs.

And Rabia al-Joburgiya (MTBBC) said: My open root chakra helps me to perform my work at a deeper level. People of Ignorance claim I cannot think straight during menses. Verily, I can keep planes from crashing into each other or judge court cases while blood flows from me. Our cycles do not cause incompetence in the work world; it's the other way around: Needs the rigid work world to become more fluid, better geared towards human cycles, male, female, mithli, khuntha, ghulamiya, mukhannath, laziza, azizatu nafsiha, hijri, mujtama' al-meem, and all genders – before it destroys the Earth and its Waters.

From the chronicles of those who read with care the Signs that emerge from Their Vaginas:

One said: I am not pregnant. What a relief. And the other said: I am not pregnant. What a sadness. And the Truthteller said: Knowledge that comes with blood, I welcome you. Help me to witness truth for my people.

And one said: I am pregnant. What a joy. And she began to dance her joy for she wanted this above all things. And another one said: I am pregnant. What a joy and a worry mixed. This will change every instant of my life to the end of my days and I am afraid it will change who I am. I need to think about this.

And one said: I am pregnant. What a disaster. I chose this Not. Horror fills me. I will remove the clot of mingled mucus/nutfah amshaj before it forms a mudghah. And she went to Nadifa the Wise Chemist and the Wise Chemist said: Yes, our science has wrought many remedies at your stage of alaqah, and the Wise Chemist gave her a remedy. And she replied:

Thank al-Raheema for providing science and remedies. And this is our heritage, though a later age will hide it.

And that particular Wise Chemist said: Know that if you wait longer, you would need the Surgeon. And know that the Surgeon of our Order will abort your clot only until the Spirit is breathed into it, one hundred and twenty days. After that, only if it were due to abomination or threatened your life. For our particular order holds the principle that the ascertained life – Yours – hath priority over potential life. And she replied: I will hurry and tell my friend who is troubled and contemplating, for she now hath but nutfah amshaj, the clot of mingled seeds.

They ask thee concerning abortion. Say, It is a difficult Blessing not to be overused.

They ask thee concerning menopause. Say, The queen unwinds her red turban, in fits and starts; roll out the polkadotted carpet. Behold, the hormone cometh – and goeth. Prepare, prepare. You are on the cusp of the Second Half of the Clamshell. Our ancestors among the Elders of Himyar and Saba, who carried in their breastbones the Wisdom of Balqis the Sceptical Thinker and Council-consulting Queen, welcomed the Second Half by distributing baskets of moisturising unguents along with calcium and hormones, from all the cable cars in their ancient cities. And the Enterer into the Age of Abundance ritually received a robe whose sleeves were embroidered with this prayer: May you remain as sprightly as Queen Balqis when She lifted her Skirts as one wading into a Lake. And on the other sleeve: May Bodilicious Life Dimensions threshold your Elder Half.

Via the khuntha Muslimah ibn Laziz, the ancient prophet and messenger Rasula bint Nabia (MRIHM – May Rahmana

Invent Her Mention) said: Behold, my period leaveth me. My blood no longer moves with the Moon-Tides. I have Ascended to the Age of Generosity. And I will wear giant turquoise flowers at my waist in celebration.

And when Bibi Sidra the Truthteller matured to the Age of Forty, she gained the clear-sightedness of Zarqa al-Yamama of yore, and left the Man Who Held Her at Bay because finally she could see that he held her at bay, and became a Truthteller. And this was her Age of Perimenopause and it was as excruciating as writhing in a birth canal as she twisted and turned; verily, Transformation is excruciating.

Then climbed She up the Mountain to the Cave and spent uncounted Epochs prayerfully Meditating. And she meditated until she passed through almost all genders, but not all, because they are beyond count. She was rocked in the waves of the Ocean of genders and became one with each wave. And she reached the Fullness of her Abundance, and she held her Arc in Abundancy for decades more, by the human way of accounting.

And one said: I have reached the Age of Fifty-three and I have lost my Libido. Where has mischievous Libido gone? And she did gird herself mightily, and chased her Lost Libido through the Bush. Until one day, she caught her Lost Libido, tied it up with twine in the boot of her car, and brought it wriggling home. And another one said: Lo, I am at Peace without my Libido and do bid it farewell; I have other Joyful Things to Do in Abundance.

And the people of Ignorance said: Menopause is Sinn al-Ya'ss, the age of despair for all hope of pregnancy is gone. These are the same people who freaked out at the person's menarche, and made to fear her monthly blood; dumb they are to the contradiction they have created, caught in its deceitful net. Nay, say it is the Age of Takrim and the Age of Abundancy.

And Sri Saudari the Shaikha of Wholesomeness said instead, via her two lifelong unmarried great-aunts, Verily and Merrily, you have entered the Age of Freedom, Age of Accolade, Age of Honouring. Sinn al-Karama, wa enti al-Mukarrama. And Our Mother Hawwa added: Honey, concoct you a jar of Vaginal lube that suits you. How doth your body?

And one said: I have a whisker where none grew before. And another one said: No one told me pussy hair goes grey too! Ya Mother Hawwa, what is the meaning of this? And this latter is narrated in multiple narrations.

How doth your body feel? One said: It thickens in Abundance, and my torso more so. And LaDawna Bint Clara al-Chicagoweeya said: This intensity comes in heated flashes, and makes me anxious and exhausted. Give me space to be this vulnerable or verily I will bite your head off. I am learning to wield my new Blessings gracefully. This process is an Abundance I will share with you.

And in another narration al-Chicagoweeya said: I need space to feel how I feel. Come not near unto me for now. But don't go too far away. And bring back leafy greens from the grocer because my body craves to restock essential nutrients. Verily, I Love the Patient Returners with Leafy Greens.

They ask Thee concerning menopause. Say, I am fucking lucky to reach it. Alive and with bodily integrity and sharp mind and healthcare access and many other privileges. Ready for mattress-shaking sex, free of the fear of pregnancy. I can wear white pants anytime now. Ready to begin exhilarating things; I am done bleeding. Almost done child-rearing. I want that last lingering child out of my house, although they are welcome back if they enter with adult shoulders and clean the inside of the microwave regularly. But with Foolishness will I no longer Abide.

And one said: I will take oestrogen and progesterone. Another one said: I will take no hormones. For People with Wombs are each a world unto themselves and each body is different. How doth your body?

Another one said: I lift weights daily to build my bones for adventures ahead. For I am looking forward to the joy of retiring and travelling the Earth and its Seas.

And another one said: I have taken a vow not to cut my hair until the tyrant is gone from my lands. For the tyrant monstrously abideth in the lands of my birth, spreading harm, his soul pulverised inside him.

How do your sweet and salt waters meet? At the Estuary, in the Flow and the Ebb? And the Truthteller (MSBSWDA – May She Be Showered with Divine Attributes) said: Warrior and Healer I have ever been in every Epoch, and I still Am, yea though I age and ache. Yea, ache I, from my inner Labia to that sinew I can't reach between my shoulder blades. A one-hour massage would be nice. Build me a heated spa. I understand Sauna now, more fully, and our bathing rituals; bring them with you. Meanwhile, I embrace this productive Ebb and the insights given to me when I look on the world from within it. Joy comes to me and I give it Room. When I feel like crying, I cry. For all that is going down in the world, for the unfulfilled promises that are detaching from their uterine walls and bleeding out. For Women and Girls and Queer Human Beings raped and knifed and battered and silenced about it. For Men and Boys and Nonbinary Human Beings gunned down whose bleeding goes unheeded. For Children growing thinner, their futures trammelled. For those under occupation, and those whose souls are occupied by evil, and those in prisons of another's making, and those in prisons of their own making. My monthly blood ebbs from me and joins the river of human blood and I am One with the Ocean. This is my prayer as my Flow Ebbs: Let the rancour bleed out of my heart but not its Tenderness.

With gratitude to the many, many whose writings cleared paths for me, including Dr Amina Wadud, Dr Sahar Amer and Dr Samar Habib.

Mohja Kahf (she/ي) has been a professor of comparative literature and Middle Eastern studies at the University of Arkansas since 1995. She is the author of a novel, three books of poetry and an academic book. Her scholarly book is *Western Representations of the Muslim Woman: From Termagant to Odalisque*. Some of her writing is available in Arabic, Turkish, Japanese, Italian, German and French translations. She is a founding member of the Radius of Arab American Writers, and the winner of a Pushcart Prize. In 2011 she joined the Syrian Nonviolence Movement (اك السلمي السوري الحر), which was founded by protest organisers inside Syria.

I CHOOSE TO BE EVERY PART OF ME

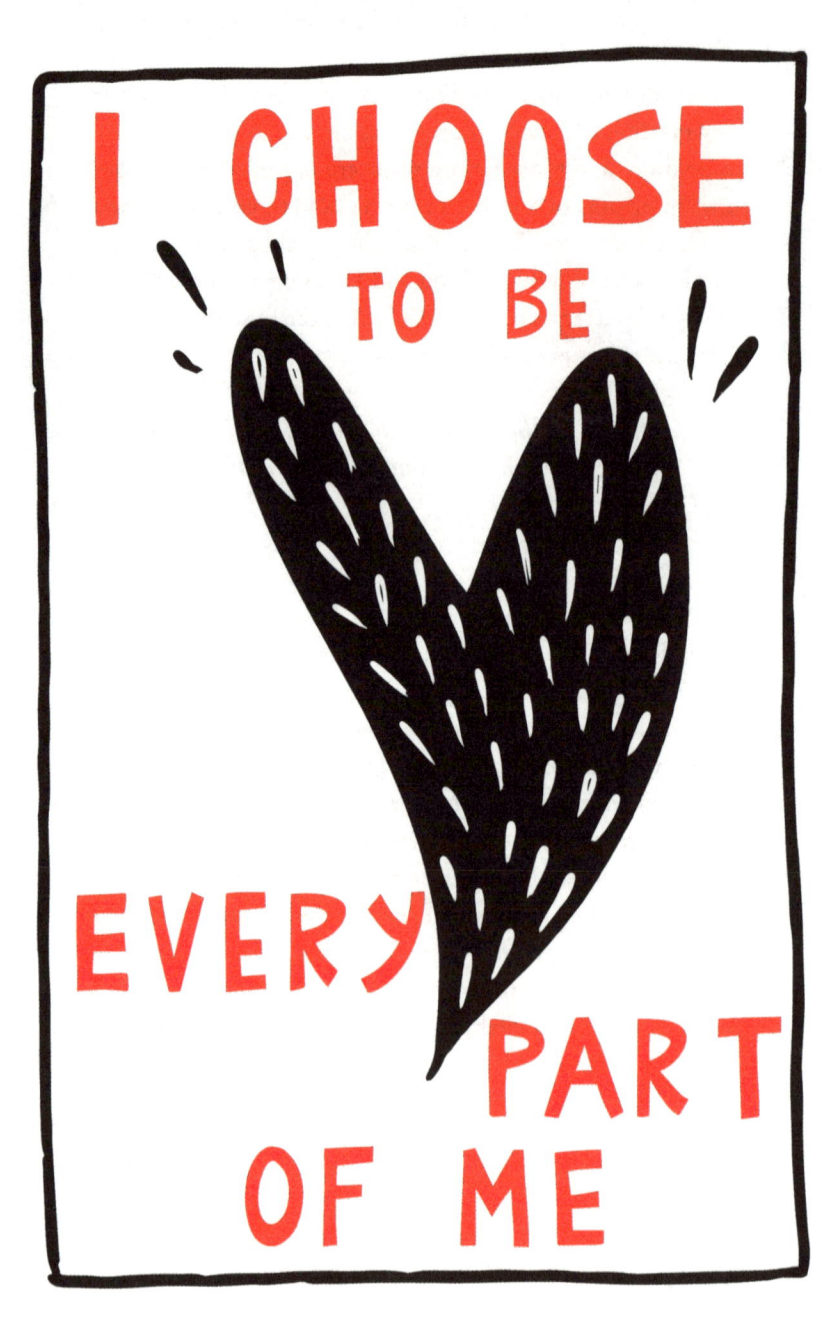

My Bleeding Life

Emmett Jack Lundberg

As a white, transmasculine person who is frequently read as cis, I am often and unusually aware of the space that I take up. While I believe this is especially helpful in understanding and being aware of my privilege, I also at times question my presence in spaces where my voice is truly important, and where I can often add an overlooked narrative.

My immediate reaction to being asked to write a piece for a book about menopause was, 'Why should my voice be a part of something that I so desperately wanted to avoid? Who am I to talk about this?' And it dawned on me that this is exactly why my voice is necessary in this space.

I started hormone replacement therapy (testosterone) at age twenty-eight, well into years of traumatic bleeding and gynaecological maladies, and long before I would have experienced my body's own time-induced disruption of bleeding. But menopause is simply defined as twelve months after your last period, and so I entered this phase just shy of my thirtieth birthday. Save for my hysterectomy surgery that caused a brief return of blood, and a spiral into dysphoria the following year.

I experienced a form of menopause that is common in trans folks on testosterone, one that often includes similar symptoms to cis women's menopausal experiences, i.e. hot flashes and weight fluctuations. It was a time of overwhelming joy for me, as most of my life, getting my period had been physically and mentally excruciating. For many years after my hysto, I was still terrified of my period returning. As if its power might transcend medical science. Writing this account is a true test in coming to terms with the history of my own body, one that is both gruelling and freeing.

From the moment I got my first period, and every month thereafter, sixteen years in total, it was a compounding trauma. Before I learned how to use a tampon, I sat in a seventh-grade science class, wearing one of those thin, crinkly track suits that were so popular in the nineties – a purple one – and bled straight through my pad and my pants, onto the plastic, beige chair. I rushed to the bathroom, tying the jacket (thank God!) around my waist. And from that moment forward, I carried the shame of visible blood, and the hope that my torturous middle-school classmates had not seen it.

Learning to use a tampon was awkward, uncomfortable and an added layer of dysphoria for me. I've never been comfortable with penetration of any kind, for pleasure or for practicality, so tampons were a new, necessary enemy. My periods were so heavy for most of my bleeding life that on heavy-flow days I would go through an ultra-plus tampon (or whatever is the heaviest/thickest) *and* a pad in just a half-hour. In my mid-twenties I sat hunched for hours overnight on the toilet while I had my period because it didn't make sense to try and change out everything and go to sleep for the very short time I had before absorption stopped.

At twenty-four I was diagnosed with a uterine fibroid that was surgically removed six months later. The doctor was focused on keeping my uterus intact for 'future fertility' reasons, but when they opened me up, the fibroid had grown to the size of a grapefruit and had obviously been causing havoc on my system. I was severely anaemic, something I had been dealing with since high school, and that still plagues me to this day. I remember the doctor being shocked that I was still standing because my iron was so low.

Subsequent diagnosis of both endometriosis and cysts on my ovaries led to a total hysterectomy two years after I started hormone replacement therapy, at age thirty. By this time, the endometriosis had spread much more than my surgeon realised and she had to call in a second surgeon while I was under anaesthesia to help remove it all. I didn't know this until a month later when I received a bill from the unknown doctor for $25,000, which was not covered by my particular insurance.

I'm convinced that this onslaught of gynaecological maladies was in direct relation to my transness. My body knew before I did that something was not right and it reminded me of that every single month for sixteen long years. I had to have the experience of bleeding to know that this experience was not mine to hold onto so tightly, but instead to be able to let go and free myself of it.

After my hysto, I had a tough recovery. I bled a lot. A lot more than I expected to and a lot more than was comfortable. It had only been a year and a half since I'd stopped bleeding because of the testosterone, but I had become so accustomed to my new reality and it felt like such incredible relief, in stark contrast to the many years that had come before.

A few weeks after my surgery, I started work on a film job that added to the stress and trauma of bleeding. I shared a direct office with about eight or ten other people, and within that bullpen office we all shared a single bathroom. So, while I was still bleeding profusely, doing my best not to have a complete breakdown from my gender dysphoria, at a job where I was not out as trans to everyone, with no on-site HR department to offer support, I had to use a bathroom in which I was convinced the crinkle of a pad wrapper could be heard like an echo through the studios. I bundled the pads up excessively in toilet paper before putting them in the open-mouthed trash can. It was probably one of the worst daily situations I've ever been in in my entire life. All of this, coupled with my attempts to put up work boundaries while starting production on my own series, led to one of my supervisors posting a job listing for my replacement without my knowledge.

For at least three to four years after my hysto, whenever I sweated too much, or peed a little, I was paranoid that my period had returned. From where, I couldn't tell you, but I was running to the bathroom to make sure, whether logic prevailed or not.

While I am writing this, I'm still to this day experiencing hot flashes. It happens if my testosterone levels dip too low or when I'm testing a new hormone-delivery method. They are a warning sign that my body is not happy or in its ideal state. And I'm reminded of how deeply uncomfortable these symptoms can be. Anyone who has to deal with this discomfort for any amount of time deserves all the space, support and resources they need to live comfortably.

For a long time I didn't want to talk about my period or when I used to bleed. I was worried that it would change people's perception of me. That somehow, while standing in front of them, ten years after starting hormone replacement therapy, the resonance of my voice or the scruff on my face would simply be erased by sharing a part of my history that is traditionally associated with a 'female' body, whatever that means. Trans folks bleed too. Nonbinary folks bleed. Trans men bleed. To bleed does not make one 'female' and to be female does not always make one bleed. Thankfully, these days, I feel a lot of pride in my lived experience. I know that every part of who I was is a part of who I am because it shaped my being. Even nine years after the last drop of blood from my hysto surgery, I can remember the sensation, the emotional state, the way it felt to bleed.

When I stopped bleeding, when I really allowed myself to know that this part of my life was over, it was a huge transformation. It allowed me a great deal of physical, emotional and mental healing. My body breathed a sigh of relief when it was given the chance to finally rebuild its stores of iron after so many years of running on empty and causing some long-term health effects. It's only in the last couple of years that I have found some relief for lifelong fatigue, shortness of breath and light-headedness. And I still always have cold hands and feet despite the rest of my body being a heater. I'm still prone to low ferritin (the protein that stores iron) and will always have to be aware of that, but I'm learning how to give my body what it needs to feel its best.

Emotionally, it's like living a different life. I don't have to feel so goddamn uncomfortable every month for what felt like perpetuity. Now that I'm well on the other side of it, I can see how traumatic this was for me. It was a painful, gushing, energy-sapping, wild, awful reminder – at least twelve times a year – of the things that my body wasn't. The things that felt out of alignment with who I was. I don't know if I'll ever be fully healed from this experience. But I'm OK with that now because of what it taught me and because it is in the past. When you're in the middle of a traumatic event, you keep going; you don't have the wherewithal to stop, take stock and let it wash over you. You can't. I can't. I'm not able to understand the depths until I'm on the safety of a new shoreline. And what I understand now is that my monthly bleeding felt like an always-present invader in my body. I knew it was there; it was just under the surface, at most only a few weeks away from its devastating return. My monthly bleeding was definitely one of, if not the worst of, my dysphoria-inducing physicalities.

I used to plan my life around my bleeding. I had to. I rarely felt up for socialising, did not feel like working (although I never had the option not to), and I definitely did not want to schedule any travel around it. It ran my life in many ways. It ran my life while it was the worst body invader I could imagine.

So you can guess how much respite I felt when I knew, really knew in my physical being, that this part of my life was over. Joy upon joy. I still feel it. I'm still so grateful for every day where I don't have to experience that kind of bleeding. It's funny, because now in conversation with my partner, whenever I mention something related to my bleeding life, they laugh a little bit and simply say, 'I forgot.' And I am able to get there too, forgetting. I can allow myself the space to let go of a lot of the heaviness, the anxiety, the dread. I won't ever truly forget it, but now I can live with it. I can live with this part of my history.

One of the best parts of being on this side of the bleeding is that it doesn't feel like it controls my life any more. It's not something I need to think about when I'm in my daily, weekly, monthly or yearly life. I can make plans. I can travel, though the ongoing Covid pandemic continues to impact all aspects of our lives, travel included. I can simply live my life without waiting for the ever-steady flow of blood on the horizon. I feel free. A deep liberation in my body and soul that didn't exist before.

In a lot of ways, it feels like I've had an experience opposite to a lot of folks who bleed. I never mourned this loss. I celebrated it. It wasn't a time of distressing physical and bodily change for me, it was a time of great excitement and newness and possibility. I finally saw my life fully in front of me, a life that was bright and liberated. What if we all experienced life's changes this way? What if we really understood the fluidity of our human experience? None of us stay the same, in any way. Each day we live, we change. It might not always be perceptible to us on a conscious level, but to live is to change. And to have a human body is to experience physical changes to that body over time, if we are lucky enough to grow old.

As I mentioned earlier, I am a white trans person. This allows me a lot of privilege that is not given to my Black, brown and other trans siblings of colour. As I write this, the United States is continuing its barrage of anti-trans legislation. The worst year in history for anti-trans legislation was 2022, and 2023 outpaced it. By othering trans folks, by putting forth legislation and op-ed pieces that serve to paint us as different in cis people's eyes, the amount of hate we are subjected to increases. Murders and brutality increase. Especially against trans women and trans femmes of colour. Multiple states in the US have already enacted bans on hormone therapy and gender-affirming care, forcing adult trans people to detransition or move. This is state-sanctioned violence. I can't be the only trans person who would rather die than detransition.

My hope in contributing to this book is to offer the other side of that coin. To show that trans folks' experiences are human experiences. That we live and breathe and experience joy and pain in the same way as our cis counterparts. The distinction between cis and trans is not actually all that much, and it should not be seen or used as a weapon between us. But if folks in power are insistent on making it a weapon, I will continue to fight for my community for as long as my physical body allows.

Trans folks have existed for all of time. Just because we now live in a time where media and ideas can be seen quickly on a global scale does not mean that the wave of emergence of trans narratives and voices is because it is a new phenomenon. We have existed alongside you forever and we are finally able to make our voices heard.

And as it goes for the cis experience, the trans experience is unique to the individual. Not every trans person who bleeds has the same fraught experience that I do or did. Some of us talk about it, some of us don't. Each and every one of us is one of a kind in every piece of the human puzzle.

I hope that we all keep talking about the hard stuff. That we keep sharing the stuff that makes us uncomfortable and ashamed. That we begin to understand how wildly different and exquisitely the same the human experience is.

I felt ashamed and didn't talk about bleeding through my pad the first time it happened to me.

I felt ashamed and didn't talk about how uncomfortable bleeding was for me.

I felt ashamed and didn't talk about how heavy bleeding was for me.

I felt ashamed and didn't talk about how uncomfortable using tampons was for me.

I felt ashamed and didn't talk about how bad bleeding was for me.

Now that I've put this piece onto paper, I can let it all go.

In the States, society at large does not want to talk about bleeding or periods or anything in relation to these things. Being a trans person on top of that makes for an incredibly challenging existence.

On the practical side, I started using restrooms labelled for 'men' early on in my transition (in truth I was being read as male before making this change), while I was still bleeding, and unlike restrooms traditionally labelled for 'women', there are no small trash receptacles in the stalls. I had to wrap up my absorbents and carry those wads out with me to the sink to throw them away. Another layer of shame.

On the emotional side, for me, it's a challenge to try and compartmentalise parts of myself. As I write this now I'm realising that this is why I feel the urge to share so many pieces of my life, because all of the many things that I experience are what make me exactly who I am. By severing different pieces of myself, I feel incomplete, not fully me. I am a trans masc person who spent many years bleeding. This is a part of who I am and it has informed the person I am today. I don't want to hide that or be ashamed of it. I want to embrace it as something that makes me uniquely me.

Menopause, like transition, I believe, is unfairly categorised (mostly by able-bodied, straight, cis, white men) as a life change that is about the destruction of something, the end of something. And to get even more explicit, menopause and the trans masculine experience are about a loss of femininity. In reality, both experiences are about creation. Creation of new ways of being, new forms of existence, new versions of ourselves. Better, more well-rounded and compassionate versions of ourselves. The most we can hope for in life is to keep learning and growing until we leave the physical plane. These, and all of our experiences, help us do that.

Life is change. If I have learned anything in almost forty years on this planet, it's that none of us stay the same in any way, shape or form. Our bodies deteriorate, our hair falls out or grows anew in unexpected places, our hair colour changes (through age or by our own hand), people we love die, we experience traumas, we create new things and people who didn't exist before. To live is to be changed by the events of your life. Whether that's menopause, transition or starting a new creative project. Every way we interact with our life changes us. And every day is a chance to change. Today I choose full integration, with all parts of myself that I have felt shame and discomfort about. I choose to own my bleeding life. I choose to be every part of me.

Emmett Jack Lundberg (he/they) is a queer and trans filmmaker, writer and actor who views the many titles he embodies as pieces of a whole that work best together. His latest feature script *This Love* (compared to Andrew Haigh's *Weekend* and Wong Kar-Wai's *Happy Together* by *The Black List*), was shortlisted by the Barnstorm Fest as one of the 150 Best Scripts of 2021. Emmett's groundbreaking series 'BROTHERS' was one of *IndieWire*'s Best of Indie TV, called 'among the boldest and frankest representations of trans male love on-screen to date' by *The Advocate*. He is a proud OUT100 Honoree and also won the Triple Threat Auteur award from the Toronto Webfest. Accolades include being a finalist in the Nashville FF Screenwriting Competition and quarterfinalist in Coppola's Zoetrope Competition. He co-edited *Finding Masculinity*, an anthology about transitioning later in life, and won his first writing award in the third grade. Hell-bent on studying and making films in NYC, he only applied to NYU's Tisch School of the Arts – early decision – and thankfully got in, spurring a lifelong love affair with New York City, no matter where he is.

I FELT LIKE
I HAD LOST
SOMETHING I HAD

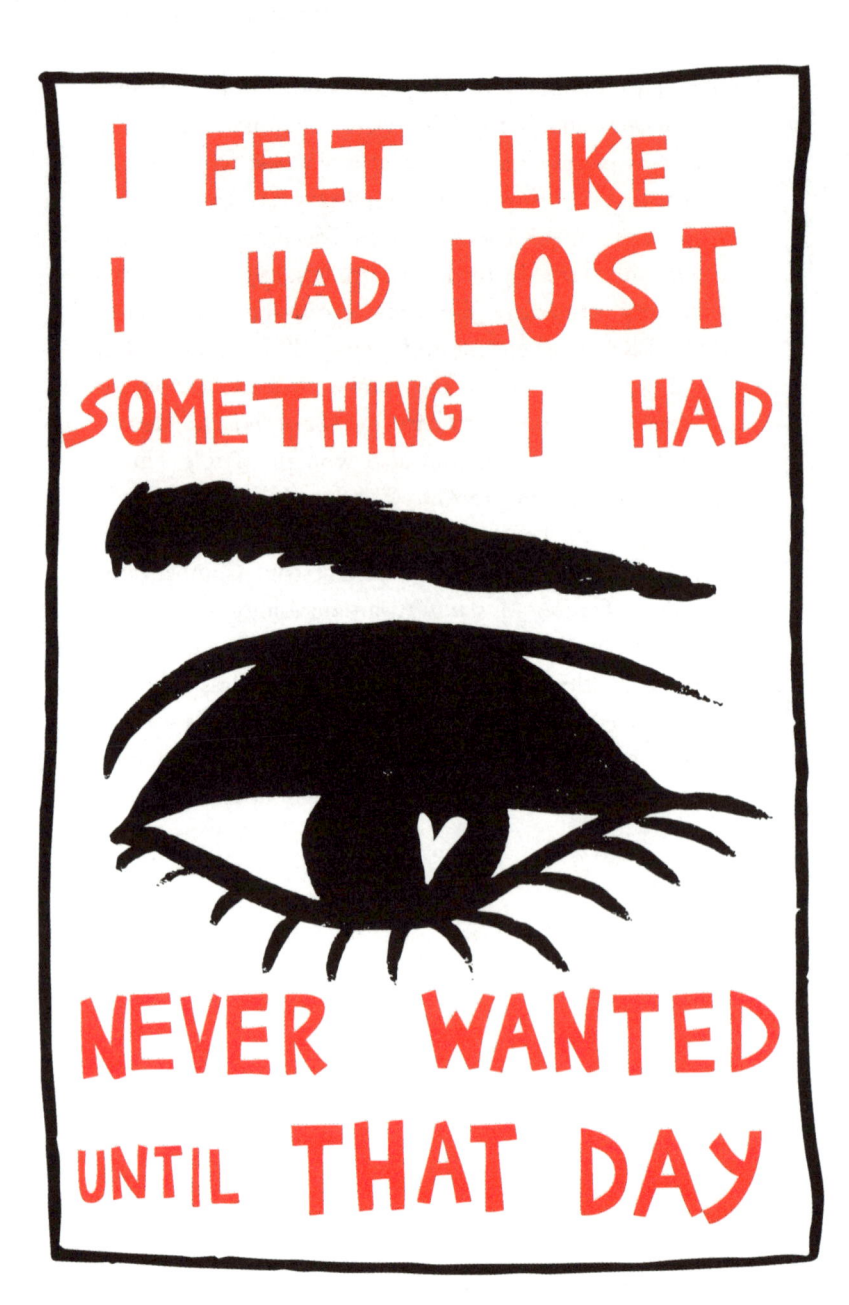

NEVER WANTED
UNTIL THAT DAY

I Don't Like Being Late: An Experience of Perimenopause From Turkey

Aslı Alpar (translated by Canan Marasligil)

It was a beautiful spring day. I went out to water the plants before the midday sun started to wither the garden. I was captivated by how the leaves were coming alive the moment water started touching the earth, when I saw my neighbour from down the street and greeted her with a smile. She slowly approached my door, asking me how I was. Just the usual neighbourly chit-chat, I thought. Until the triviality of our conversation suddenly turned into the 'child' topic.

Her boundless curiosity, which started with the question 'Can't you have children?', accrued into an overwhelming staccato of unsolicited and harassing flow of information and advice which I had great difficulty stopping. It went from how challenging it was to get pregnant in later life, to her daughter-in-law's situation, who at her late age could only get pregnant with treatment, all the way to me: that I should see a doctor as soon as possible to have my egg count checked.

In Turkey, the cultural etiquette deems such inquisition as 'normal'.

If your assigned gender is female, especially if you have a regular or formal relationship with a person whose assigned gender is male, such questions are directed at you as a 'well-intentioned warning'.

INVISIBILITY, DISCRIMINATION AND VIOLATION OF RIGHTS IN THE EXAMINATION ROOM

I am writing this essay at the age of thirty-six. Two years ago, I was diagnosed with early menopause: persistent headaches, insomnia, anxiety disorder, hot flashes and menstrual irregularity.

The Covid-19 pandemic measures were still in place in Turkey at the time, in parallel with unabated political and economic turmoil. Although I believed that what I was experiencing was mostly psychological, I still decided to remain cautious and went to the gynaecologist without waiting for my routine check-up.

In some hospitals in Turkey, gynaecology units are literally called 'Women and Birth Clinic', which is the equivalent of the 'Obstetrics and Gynaecology Clinic'. I made an appointment at a polyclinic with this name.

I will come back to my consultation palaver, but first I must state this: during gynaecology examinations in Turkey, women, intersex people and trans men are very often exposed to methods and practices in which patients' rights are ignored. The various forms of discrimination that can occur are sometimes due to the heterosexist and binary gender-based medical education, and sometimes due to the moralistic and reactionary beliefs of some doctors. Serious violations of rights are commonplace in the examination room, such as forced deprivation of reproductive autonomy, doctors who do not want to examine trans women who have completed their transition procedure, violating the rights of individuals to their own bodily autonomy, or gynaecologists who condemn unmarried women who are sexually active.

If you are a lesbian or a bisexual woman, you will be made to become completely invisible during a gynaecology exam. Part of the procedure is to ask the patient if they are sexually active, but due to cultural norms, doctors ask, 'Are you married?' When most feminists, women's or LGBTQI+-rights advocates answer this question with, 'I am not married, but I am sexually active,' because sexuality is only associated with heterosexuality, the concern always comes down to whether one wants pregnancy or not and what contraceptive one uses.

In our book *Jinekolog Muhabbetleri* (*Conversations at the Gynaecologist*),[2] which compiles a series of experiences of people who have been through discriminatory practices during a gynaecology examination, as well as from expert doctors in the field, Ayşe shares her experience: 'I've been told it was my time, that everything was in place for me to have dozens of babies. I immediately responded that I would marry my partner and crack on with it, which delighted the doctor. I even got suggestions regarding contraception. I am thirty-six years old, and very few people around me know that I am a lesbian.'

NO HEALTH INFORMATION, ONLY REPRODUCTIVE IMPOSITION!

Let me go back to the examination room where I was diagnosed with early menopause. As a bisexual woman and a right-to-health activist, I remain alert and vigilant when it comes to discrimination during gynaecology examinations. I am now used to doctors' disapproving comments expressed in their *estağfurullah* whether I mention a female partner, in answer to a question out of curiosity rather than a need to know my medical history, or when I went for a pap smear test when I was single and was asked by the doctor if 'my family knew I was doing such things'.

So this time, I entered the gynaecology examination as a married woman, making sure my bisexual identity remained invisible. Once my medical history reporting was done, I settled into the examination chair. During the ultrasound check, the doctor exclaimed, 'Aaaa!' in astonishment. The alarming interjection was followed by a, 'It's too early, your ovarian reserve is about to run out.' Which then turned into a repetition of the initial medical-history questioning: 'Are you married?'

'I am sexually active.'

'Then you immediately have to stop contraception.'

I did not respond for a while to the doctor's assumption that my partner was a cisgender male and that I wanted to reproduce, then said, 'I don't want to have children.'

The doctor, who was looking at me from the top of her glasses, pointed at me to look at the ultrasound screen, where I could only discern some dark spots, and from what I recall, these statements started pouring all over me: 'Look, these are your eggs, even though you are in the ovulation period now, they are very few' . . . 'You will regret it later. My advice is to stop contraceptives immediately' . . . 'It will be very difficult to get pregnant for you even with IVF' . . . 'You must have a child' . . .

We left the examination table and went back into the office. She sent me off, saying that I had to come back to the clinic on the third day of my period because my hormones had to be checked, and that I should take this time to think thoroughly about my situation.

Before you know it, I was back in the examination room to show the test results I gave on the third day of my period. The doctor, grimacing at my results, asked if there was any family history of early menopause. My grandmother was diagnosed with perimenopause in 1962 at the age of thirty-seven and gave birth to my mother following the treatment recommendation she got at the time. My grandmother's early menopause was, in a sense, the reason for my existence.

Then the doctor, who said that my lab values were very 'bad' for my age, commanded me, without even asking if I wanted to have a child or not, to 'stop contraception right now' and added, 'Let's plan your reproductive treatment.' Giving birth was not among my plans; I had neither the financial nor moral strength to take care of a child; I did not want to have a baby. I told the doctor. I got an insistent and intrusive response: 'Listen, my dear, you will regret it, trust me.' While she was patronising me, I was thinking that I was too young to experience menopause, that I would age prematurely, that my bones would melt following heart disease, that my face would quickly wrinkle, that sweating and insomnia would never end. I asked if there was a cure for premature menopause. She casually mentioned hormone therapies only to add that once I started these, I could never get pregnant again. She then linked my unwillingness to have children to an unhappy marriage. 'Is it your husband who doesn't want it?' she said, then, unsatisfied, rephrased the question: 'What if your spouse wants children?' (Don't you worry – I did retort, 'Let him give birth, then.')

Each of my questions regarding my health came instantly back to pregnancy. I left that examination room as an 'old' woman. At the cashier where I went to make the payment, near the 'GYNAECOLOGY AND OBSTETRICS' sign, I saw that there was a place for taking pictures with blue ornaments on the left and pink ornaments on the right. Right next to me, I saw two pregnant women, and women walking out the door with diaper bags in their hands. I felt like I had lost something I had never wanted until that day; I felt sick; I felt alone.

As if that wasn't enough, the hospital corridors were all adorned with IVF (in vitro fertilisation) ads, with pictures of happy mothers with their babies in their arms. There was not one informative poster about HPV (human papillomavirus), menstruation or how to maintain your sexual health. 'Women's disease' and obstetrics clinics do not cover people who have a womb but are not women; I learned again that in this commercialised, sexist, heteronormative and binary health system, a woman who will not give birth is not worth anything. Feminist gynaecologists and doctors who value and apply ethical principles do exist, but it is this system that makes us sick, that abandons us . . . And it is very big.

WOULD I REGRET IT?

I have dived into the first part of my process at length, now I will take you through the next two years. Four different doctors, more blood tests, but the answers and reactions I got remained the same. Only now they started calling it perimenopause instead of early menopause.

I knew it was a possibility because I work in the field of women's health, yet no doctor has provided me with the information that I could freeze my eggs. No one mentioned there were other options than giving birth to become a parent. Not a single doctor asked if I thought about pregnancy at all, and they kept assuming that my partner was a cisgender male. No doctor explained to me what hormonal therapy entailed; not only did they all recommend IVF, they never recommended any treatment that would reduce the difficult symptoms that were negatively affecting my life. I struggled with perimenopause symptoms for another year and a half. Also, I was now facing a new series of dilemmas: Did I want to have a child? Would I regret not having one? Why didn't I want one? How come these words repeated every time by a doctor, 'you will regret it', circled back to make me doubt? Me, of all people, who has been thinking about this very topic for such a long time, reading about it and even banging on about it with my peers? To cut it short: I was constantly manipulated about an unplanned and unwanted pregnancy, but I could not find any information about the treatment to replace the hormones I lost with the presumed early menopause. I even received information about the birth package, but not once did I learn anything regarding my own health. I won't even mention the risks of hormonal therapy in early menopause, or the experimental 'treatments' that have been administered to earlier generations before us.

WE ARE NOT ALONE!

I shared my journey into perimenopause and the problems I had with reproductive-focused 'women's health' experts in an article on the LGBTQI+ rights platform KaosGL.org, where I work as a journalist. Many messages and emails followed its publication. Leaving the 'Get well soon' or 'Congratulations' aside, I received similar testimonies from so many people that I decided it was important to share their views, with their consent, in this essay.[3]

I would like to remind you that the purpose of my sharing these testimonials is to reveal and denounce a common problem: namely, the existence of health policies focusing on reproduction rather than our health and needs. And I would like to underline that the problem is systemic, and that many doctors do adhere to professional ethics without violating patients' rights. To sum it up, those who experience early menopause say the following: We consult a health institution with a specific health problem, they come up with a diagnosis, but we are not adequately informed about the process. The information is focused on our capability for getting pregnant. We have no idea about what awaits us in the process.

Testimony 1
'It's as if they were more concerned with my unborn child than with my health.'

From my first visit, doctors kept saying similar things they had told you: 'If you were married' ... 'If you had frozen your eggs' ... 'You can still freeze them, but there will be a need for hormonal load, there are risks' ... Doctors whose office walls are full of pictures of babies. I was even told: 'You can buy eggs from Cyprus'! It was as if they were more concerned with my unborn child than with my health. It was my body that we were making decisions about. Shouldn't it be ensured that I understand my situation and what is at stake so that I am given all the necessary information to make a decision myself?

Testimony 2
'I still don't know what I will face when I enter menopause.'
I would like to share my experience as someone who has been dragged in and out of obstetrics clinics since I was nine years old, how I had been under incredible pressure to freeze my eggs because my last egg reserve was low. First of all, almost all health centres do embryo freezing, but only a few do egg freezing. I only found one hospital in a big city like İzmir. Then the government allows them to stay frozen for five years. After that, you need to get a special permit for each additional year, which is very difficult to get from the Ministry of Health. Not to mention that we are being exposed to and triggered by slogans such as: 'We can provide virginity reports, don't you worry'! Instead of informing you, doctors just try to start the procedure directly, adding psychological distress to an already difficult situation. The government certainly doesn't pay for it. Unfortunately, egg freezing is yet another challenge women are facing in our country. I needed

to go through surgery, but it was risky. They put this risk aside and instead obsessively focused on the possibility that I may not have any eggs left after the surgery. When I decided not to freeze my eggs and went to see my doctor again, I was told that I would enter menopause in a short time, and that the problem I was experiencing (endometriosis) would disappear when I entered menopause, so there was no need for a risky surgery. I still don't know what to expect when I reach menopause. I am sharing my experience everywhere I can. We have to talk about this.

Testimony 3
'Would it cause any problems?'
I learned that my egg reserves were about to run out. Good to know, but I had no idea what to do next! IVF treatment was recommended; I was given time to think. I was told that if I delayed the decision-making, I was about to enter a road of no return. I learned almost everything there was to know about IVF treatment. Would it cause any problems? Nobody told me anything besides concerns regarding pregnancy. I received no information regarding hormonal treatment; it's as if all the information routes were made to lead to contraception or reproduction, nothing else.

MENOPAUSE BEYOND THE EXAMINATION ROOM

So, how was my perimenopausal status received within my social circles and work life?

It is important to highlight that my experience does not reflect everyone else's, yet I am drawing from it to describe perceptions related to women's health in our society. Ever since I discovered I was bisexual – almost two decades ago – I have been a part of queer solidarity. I am one of the people fighting for the queer feminist transformation of health policies stemming from the field I work in. I work in one of the few institutions that regulate menstrual leave in working life in Turkey. After receiving my perimenopause diagnosis, I have contributed work on 'menopause leave', which will regulate the working hours, if needed, during the processes of early menopause, menopause and surgical menopause within my institution. My partner has been my best supporter during my perimenopause process. For these reasons, I did not experience the views society has on menopause within my close circles.

Where I live, women who enter menopause are prone to be abandoned by their husbands because they are regarded as 'no longer productive'. Menopause may be considered shameful, and the effects of menopause in working life can be ignored, while women in the menopausal process may be mocked and excluded from social life. In addition, menopause is only associated with cisgender women. Trans men with a uterus and ovaries tend to avoid health institutions for fear of discrimination during their menopausal process, and therefore are pushed into experiencing it on their own. This may lead to an increase in health issues that can cause serious harm. Discussing menopause is not a popular topic, even within the LGBTQI+ community. Although male gay domination within the queer movement has shifted a lot in the last decade, the menopause of bisexual and lesbian women, intersex or trans men has not entered regular discourse yet.

WORD OF MOUTH

Let's also look at some figures reflecting the general framework in Turkey:

- There is not a single mention of menopause in the Turkish Labor Law No. 4857, which regulates work.
- In 2022, men killed at least 327 women and inflicted violence on 793 women in Turkey.[4]
- Turkey's LGBTQI+ rights record is also quite bad. In ILGA-Europe's* 'Annual Review of the Human Rights Situation of LGBTI People in Europe and Central Asia', Turkey received 4 points out of 100 for LGBTQI+ rights, ranking 48th among 49 European countries.[5]
- Turkey ranks 129th out of 146 countries in the 2022 Gender Gap Index of the World Economic Forum.[6]
- The Council of Europe Convention on Preventing and Combating Violence Against Women and Domestic Violence (aka the Istanbul Convention), which entered into force on 1 August 2014 in Turkey and eleven European countries, was unlawfully terminated in Turkey on 20 March 2020 by presidential decree.

In addition to these figures, public officials, who are also responsible for protecting the rights of women and LGBTQI+

---

* According to their website, ILGA-Europe are an independent, international, non-governmental umbrella organisation uniting over 700 organisations from fifty-four countries across Europe and Central Asia.

communities, often produce misogynistic, homophobic and biphobic as well as transphobic discourses and policies. Under such circumstances we can conclude that the process of menopause in Turkey is being pushed into word-of-mouth practices up to the point of becoming totally invisible.

The reproductive health policies of the twenty-year rule of President Erdoğan's Islamic political Justice and Development Party (AKP) are aimed at the promotion of reproduction and not at all of sexual rights. Access to contraceptive methods has been made more difficult. Although abortion has been a legal right since 1983, in reality it is not being practised due to reactionary pressures on hospitals and doctors.[7] Within this political atmosphere, which I have tried to summarise, it would not be erroneous to say that, as a result of outdated policies, menopause feels like the 'finish line' for women, whose value in society is being reduced to motherhood. In this political arena, just as has been happening to menstruation, women's sexuality and puberty, menopause has become an unspeakable topic. While the feminist movement and the LGBTQI+ community continue to exist under the systematic attacks of the government, there remains little opportunity to focus on producing any kind of discourse or policy around menopause. For hundreds of thousands of women, menopause becomes an experience in which they are mostly invisible, a process in which they are subjected to misogyny-based mockery and all kinds of discrimination.

On one of the nights I was hit with insomnia, one of the first symptoms of perimenopause, I started browsing my library and came across a poetry collection by Nilgün Marmara. The following lines of her poem titled 'Body' reflected my inner emotions of what it means to be experiencing menopause in Turkey:

> Your body is a tower.
> The steps inside are manifold, dark and humid.
> You climb up in laughter,
> Come down in cries![1]

Every single period of our life is precious. I invite us all to continue to resist so that we do not have to cry, whether we are climbing up or coming down, so that we are never left alone in our experiences.

One more thing I would like to share before I end my essay. In the first month of 2023, I got pregnant without going through any treatment, despite the levels of my early-menopause hormones. I did not want to go on with the pregnancy and terminated it. And to the neighbour I wrote about in the beginning of my story who asked me, 'Can't you have children?' I replied, 'Indeed, I cannot have children.' My sweet menopause, you have already given me courage.

Aslı Alpar (she/her) was born in 1987 in Ankara. She is an illustrator and journalist. She graduated from the University of Istanbul's Department of Public Finance in 2008. In 2018, Aslı completed an MA in women's studies. Since 2016, she has been organising queer cartoon workshops in various cities across Turkey, aiming to increase the number of works that highlight gender equality and diversity in cartooning.

Canan Marasligil (she/they) is a multilingual writer, artist and literary translator based in Amsterdam. Canan publishes a newsletter and podcast titled *The Attention Span*, where they can take the time to reflect, to analyse and to imagine our societies through writing, art and culture. cananmarasligil.net

This Is Going Somewhere Good

Ann Marie McQueen

It started happening one night this winter, on my back on a yoga mat in front of the television, having just completed one of the yin classes that help me sleep.

I thought about one of the worst (and most pivotal) nights of my life; I had not in a while. After 9/11, at thirty-one, and while working as the sole City Hall reporter for the *Ottawa Sun*, the tabloid paper in Canada's capital, I decided I needed to travel. The ten days I had spent visiting a friend in London in the mid-nineties, with a surprise venture to Glastonbury (hello Johnny Cash, Björk and Blind Melon), and party trips to Cancún, Puerto Plata and Fort Lauderdale didn't count.

And I was about as un-savvy a traveller as you could get.

I had a money belt, Triple A travel insurance, a suitcase with no wheels, no coat (it was December) and a Eurail pass. Among the errors I would make on that trip: booking into a Christian hostel in Amsterdam because a friend had stayed there (it had a curfew! And proselytisers! And no alcohol!); leaving my passport on a check-in desk in Berlin Central

Station, only to hear a name being called over the loudspeaker many, many, many times, until I realised it was mine tangled up in that German accent; and spending too much platonic time in France with a guy who only talked about his ex-girlfriend from three years prior.

A person who I didn't spend enough time with? The handsome Frenchman a waiter had mischievously sat beside me in a 4th arrondissement café by Notre-Dame. After chatting haltingly through our meals in a mix of his English and my French, we walked to the metro and stared longingly at each other for several seconds. I turned away, though, strangely cautious for me, and it was because of what had happened the first night in Paris.

And that is what I remembered at fifty-two, almost fifty-three, on the floor of my apartment in Abu Dhabi.

Full of excitement to have finally taken the plunge (and the vacation days) to travel, I went to the Eiffel Tower and then wandered across the Seine to the Trocadéro (as, for sure, a guidebook told me to). As I often did in those days, I smoked a Du Maurier Light king size as I stared across at the lights on that sparkly global landmark, taking in all the people around me, marking a moment of extreme wonder. I felt then, as I often did in those days, on the precipice of greatness.

I usually wished there was someone to share such moments with – being single was hard at the turn of the millennium (I have a lot to compare it to, having *never married*). It was the age of 'baby panic', and I had been dating unsuccessfully for three years since my last relationship, much longer than I'd figured it would take after I'd ended a relationship destined for marriage for . . . more. Everyone was getting married and having kids. But I didn't feel any of that as I inhaled the delicious, meaningful cigarette, and promised myself I would always travel, even if it was alone. Because I now knew, firsthand, that it was everything.

I got up full of hope and happiness, blissfully unaware of my surroundings, leaving a platform filled with people and almost skipping down a set of stairs. I kept descending even as my brain registered a group of young men on the landing below, eight or nine of them. I heard one of them say something to the others. There was a second before they surrounded me, when I pictured myself being more careful.

But then a hand slapped down over my mouth, and they were pulling at me from all directions. Having been kickboxing four or five days a week, I was strong, and had picked up valuable self-defence tips from my instructor, who was a jiujitsu master. (I liked to joke with my friends that I could throw down with anyone, provided there was music playing, we all faced a mirror and punched in unison.)

It was a few years after the American security expert Gavin de Becker had done the rounds promoting his 1997 book *The Gift of Fear*, and I'd seen him on *The Oprah Winfrey Show*. His top piece of advice? Fight to the death not to leave the initial scene of an attack, because if that happened, it was usually too late.

All of these things were in my mind when I somehow dropped down in the middle of them; hunched and curled up on the ground, elbows close, hands high, protecting my face and my core. I kicked and kicked, hearing grunts as my feet made contact. I could feel my ridiculous money belt being pulled out and snapping back under my shirt. The hand kept coming for my mouth, but he could never clamp back on.

And when they had given up and run away, I literally came to lying on my back and kicking the air, tasting blood in my mouth and realising the hysterical top-volume staccato screaming I'd heard the entire time had been coming from me, so loud it had attracted a crowd of people up above.

There's some more fun stuff. Like the American ladies who, when I yelled, 'HOLY CRAP!' responded in a drawl, 'Are you from America, sweetheart?' and then, 'Hold on, we're coming down to get you.'

The six Heinekens I later downed at the hostel's bar after they'd delivered me; polishing off the rest of the Du Maurier Lights; the insane feeling of being jacked up on adrenalin for hours; and a drunken Brit with gross hair and very bad teeth who'd been increasingly concerning in the hostel bar. And who later – still, I wonder how – managed to stick his foot in the door of my room when I finally tried to retire in the wee hours, whipping out his dick and peeing in my garbage can before I screamed at him to get out, and then proceeded to wander the halls bellowing, keeping us all awake.

I immediately parsed that *very bad night* for myself and others. It was *a story*.

I even added schtick about how I was able to fight them off despite not having music and an instructor and a mirror. I cannot remember ever crying about it; just yuck-yucking like I was the main character in a romantic comedy filled with hilarious mayhem and mishaps.

It had been like that for almost twenty-two years – it was like that with most of my pain, let's be honest – until I did yin yoga, and started remembering for real, and for the first time relived those moments as they actually felt: like I was fighting for my life, and it was not at all funny. The feeling bubbled up out of my knees and hips, from my back and around my ears and my throat.

And I cried so hard and for so long I felt like I might choke.

When it was over, my cat Ninja Jr was sitting on my chest purring, and I was sniffling and doing those two quick-breaths that happen after a Big Cry, and I let myself accept how scary and awful an experience it had been.

I came together in some major way that night. Something clicked, I embodied myself, and I let go. The distance between what happened to me and how I felt about it shrank wildly.

That was sometime in February, around the time that my gynaecologist noted I hadn't had a period in almost six months. I think that period was my last, but who knows, in this epic perimenopause that's been going on for more than a decade. It came out of nowhere after four months of nothing, a brilliant, bright-red, seven-full-days, no-cramps affair that felt to me like no other period I'd had. It hit, in every way, like one last blaze of fertile glory. I've felt myself ovulating only once since, months later, and it was also profound, pronounced perfection, complete with firing on all cylinders, heightened senses, fiery libido and those one-sided lower abdominal pains I found out from a nurse friend were called *Mittelschmerz*, which is German for 'middle pain'.

At one point I texted my younger boyfriend, who lives in a different city: 'I think you could come here and get me pregnant today.' He replied: 'Do you want to?' (Gotta love a hopeful man, ready to attempt the impossible procreation we joke about all the time at the drop of a message.)

As I've moved into what I'm calling my second *menomester*, the months I need to go until 'one year without a period' marks the millisecond of menopause before postmenopause begins, I'm being overtaken by a lifting, the sense of some sort of acceleration in my own awakening. The crying about that night in Paris was just the start; and the way I was able to reframe that memory and truly process it for the first time, and then let it go out of me, has continued furiously ever since.

Somewhere around that time I read Alexandra Pope and Sjanie Hugo Wurlitzer's book *Wise Power: Discovering the Liberating Power of Menopause to Awaken Authority, Purpose and Belonging*. The Red School* founders and menstruality educators speak a language few do in this transition, and I found myself unfurling and leaning into whatever is happening – getting and giving myself full permission for all of it – as I turned each page.

I've never been in tune with my monthly cycle, other than to note that sometimes I felt horridly upset and other times on top of the world, and just as I was feeling sad about it, they said not to; that menopause provided another, last chance. They gave me permission for my sudden hermit-like inclination, where I didn't want to go anywhere or be with anyone, or even do much of anything. They said it was *essential*. They wrote about the vulnerability I felt as if they were feeling it too: the sense that my skin was thin as paper, that everything was loud, and crazy, and intrusive. They wrote about illumination, the return of light; about vital rest and repair, 'a new deep, sacred negotiation' with myself, and then revelation: 'Like a heat-seeking missile, your soul is on a

---

* See their website for more information about the organisation: www.redschool.net

mission to dock you deeply back into the root system of yourself, which holds great goodness.' And with those words, for the first time in my life I could finally believe, after so long trying, that 'great goodness' was, indeed, in me – where it had always been.

I found myself starting to almost vibrate with the knowingness of it all. My purpose, my clarity, my sense of wellness – it's all there again, but new, shiny and wonderfully sharp. It has to be truth now, or I cannot stand it.

I find myself remembering painful things when I'm listening to music full blast – something I've also started doing again in recent months – and then just shaking all of my body as I cry it out. I'm not even really sad as I'm crying, just witnessing; sorting memories like some sort of freeing factory, separating out the shame and replacing it with grace and compassion for all my past selves.

I've found myself leaving long, deeply personal, totally unexpected (by me) comments on social media posts. They could look like the ramblings of a deranged middle-aged woman, if you are the judgemental sort, but people keep liking them, sometimes weeks later. And anyway, the only thing I need to know is that they are part of all of this too, sudden reality nuggets dropped as I find my way home.

Take one request for stories of food addiction. Journals I kept in my twenties are filled with WeightWatchers tabulations, fitness plans and self-disgust of the 'I can't believe I ate four Snickers bars today' variety. I have a distinct memory of standing at my kitchen counter back when I was paying dues at my first gruelling daily-newspaper job. I don't know what was wrong, only that I downed an entire row of Premium Plus crackers, each smeared with Kraft smooth peanut butter, methodically and quickly chewing and smearing and chewing and smearing.

It's a memory I've only let myself look at as the light has returned, and it prompted this unplanned – and unstoppable – outpouring:

> I was a binge eater and started growing out of it in my thirties when I began learning about emotions, etc. But I never really thought of it – or myself – in that way (although I sure felt all the shame) until recently. It started when I was a kid: I once ate the ¾ of a container of Duncan Hines chocolate frosting that was in our fridge and then was so ashamed I took my allowance and got another one at the store and ate ¼ to make it look the same and put it back in the fridge, and then the next day my mom said, 'It looks like someone ate all the Duncan Hines frosting and then opened a new one and then ate some to make it look like the same container.' (She never missed a trick; moms never do.) And we all just stayed silent. It was the seventies, and they didn't know, but it sure would have been nice and saved me a lot of shame if someone just said, 'Hey, why'd you eat all the frosting? Were you sad? That must have made you feel sick. Next time you can talk about it.' And maybe a hug. ♡

There's no one else to talk to about it now; my mom died in 1997 and I'm not going to mention it to my dad. He turns eighty this year and doesn't need to feel bad about anything. This is about me: about deep pain, embarrassment, and self-loathing that I shuddered at and hid from for decades. I never told anyone I ate the frosting. And I never wondered why I did that, or why I – a baker from a young age – used to come home from school and mix up a bowl of raw cookie dough to quickly devour before anyone else got home. That chubby little girl has been seen, and the hurt she felt dislodged; it's through, and it's out.

I left a succinct saga on Chris Williamson's page, a former cast member on the British reality show *Love Island* turned YouTuber, podcaster and club promoter. In a clip he spoke about 'involuntary childlessness' in women, breaking it down into 10 per cent who didn't want kids, 10 per cent who couldn't have them, and the rest who failed due to 'life circumstances' (complete with air quotes). He described women in their forties suddenly realising they'd left it too late, having to go to support groups and grieve 'the family they never had'. While grumpy at the 'ooooops!' way he had generalised, I realised also maybe he was scared he'd never be able to find someone to do it all with either. And I knew exactly how that felt.

It rushed over me: how hard it was to celebrate everyone else's happiness, over and over, expensively, aggressively, at a parade of weddings and baby showers and bachelorettes spanning decades, turning my dating life into *enterpainment* for others, telling myself it was fine, and getting on with my life, but deep down believing what somehow was instilled around the time of the Duncan Hines incident: that there was something terribly wrong with me.

And I broke free of it in the time it took me to leave this:

> It's a lot more complicated than 'leaving it too late to find a partner' ... I always had partners, and dated,

and boyfriends, and looked, but none of them made me want to say, 'Yes, *YOU* can be the father of my children.' I just couldn't do it. And I'm sad about it, but I don't regret it. Being stuck with any of those guys, if I'd settled, would have not been good. Now if I could go back in time and value myself more, date different people – that I'd do! Other than that, I'm fifty-two and don't need a support group. I get sad about this, and probably always will. And it's been a very good and exciting life and I can't see how I would have done much differently because it all brought me here and maybe I was never meant to be a mother in the traditional way anyway. It's complicated, lol.

Change is like that: glacial, then all at once. Menopause, it turns out, is about exponential growth. A lifetime of badly categorised memories is moving through me swiftly, releasing in pieces so markedly and leaving me so increasingly unburdened that I feel like checking the ground around me as I walk, a bit like that time I lost seventeen pounds during a thirty-day hot-yoga challenge.

It's a sharp contrast to my wonderful, terrible forties, trying to live it up in between wandering from doctor to doctor, going to the ER for possible heart attacks and blinding headaches; the panic attacks, the whooshing feeling in my head that always made me wonder if I was going to drop out of my office chair on deadline with an aneurysm; the constant feeling and worry that I was somehow dying; the heaviness of waking in the night, lonely and low, and the morning dread that hit after I opened my eyes, giving me a snatched second of peace to compare it to; the sudden fear of flying and the recurrent nightmares, where I'd wake on my hands and knees, rummaging wildly through my bedside-table drawer looking for non-existent pills I dreamed I needed to stay alive; anxiety so bad I felt like I was levitating; a lifetime of escapist weekend partying that morphed into unpredictable blackouts; and the life collapse six years ago where I got closer to planning how to kill myself than I care to admit.

No one connected the dots, and it took until forty-seven to finally clock that it was – and had been – perimenopause. That was a relief, for sure, but I couldn't find any good information, nothing I could relate to, not even from doctors and certainly not from the media or social media. And so I pivoted and decided to launch an entire platform that would use my skills to deliver to other people the clarity, guidance, research, depth and hope that I had needed. In that work with Hotflash Inc* I found a beautiful community of people around the world, all of us at some stage of the ultimate Hero's Journey of the menopause transition, making it through more dark nights of the soul than we can count. And slowly I've started to feel a lot less alone.

After all this time slogging, *doing the work* and taking what felt like three steps forward and just as many back, I know there is more than just light at the end of this tunnel. Soberly staring down the actual barrel of menopause, fully in my body, I can finally, finally, *finally* see the other side: more free, more coherent and more me – more Ann Marie *fucking* McQueen – than I have ever been.

---

* The Hotflash Inc weekly research letter was launched in June 2020 to cover the latest clinical studies, treatments, products, guidance and more.

Ann Marie McQueen is an independent digital journalist, podcaster, and former national columnist who has split her career between North America and the Middle East and currently lives in Abu Dhabi. She has 30 years of experience in reporting, much of it focused on science, health care, health and wellness. An early adopter and disruptor, throughout her career she has worked on a variety of launches, including a newspaper, a health and wellness website, a podcast and finally, her own platform. In 2020, she founded Hotflash Inc to provide evidence, expert and experienced-based information, context and strategy for people going through perimenopause, menopause and midlife. She takes no sides in her work, searching only for the true truth among competing narratives. She does this work through her Substack newsletter, weekly podcast and a range of social media, serving a fast-growing community of more than 50,000 women worldwide. She loves plants, books, sunshine and cats.

IT HAS TO BE THE TRUTH NOW, OR I CANNOT STAND IT

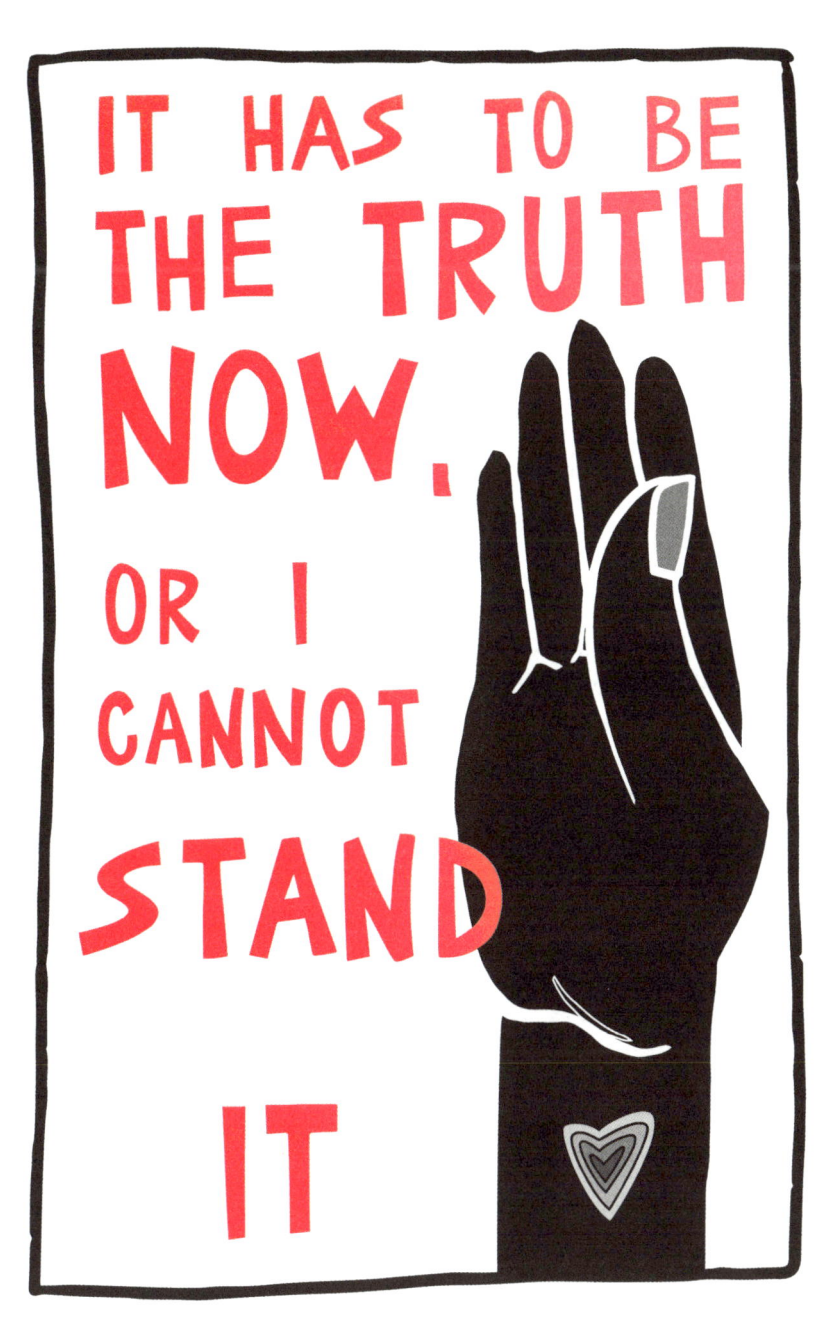

The Body Changes: Menopause Brings Change

Kimberly Dark

Being young and fat should be easy; it's hard because people hate fat without even looking closely and taking in the beauty of abundance. A pudgy girl is cute like nobody's business. A chubby adolescent looks like springtime and she's probably strong and limber and smells like the grassy hills she's been rolling down with her friends. Sunshine sits on her skin like royalty because she's the shiniest throne. She's the luminous pearl in the sand, and joy comes to all who find her. No, seriously. There's not a thing wrong with being a skinny girl. Goodness knows there's magnificence in angles, in arms akimbo, in the miracle of a body that looks like it could fold into a hundred shapes and stretch even longer than it looks. All of the bodies of girls are good bodies. Every one of them I could describe with joy and kindness.

It's not easy being any kind of a girl. The comparisons with so-called better bodies begin with our breathing, and the models for perfection aren't even human. They are airbrushed and stretched out and nipped in and whiter, with bigger eyes and lips than a human could have. Even the bodies that get praise also hear warnings. Don't get fat, don't be a slut, don't dress like that, look like that, whatever you do.

I was a fat girl and then a fat young adult and now, fat and postmenopausal. I was taught to look at bodies in the same ways as everyone else, but I learned to overcome that programming. It's more accurate to say that the programming is still inside me, but I added to it. I added an ability to look and not critique, to observe, understand and appreciate. At the beginning, though, I learned the rules like a religious text, and attended modelling-school training when I was eight. I knew bigger is badder and wiggles are wrong, and strength, well, who cares about that unless you're on a rugby team. Which would be bad. Being compared to an ox or a moose or a buffalo is not a good thing when you're a girl.

I'm sure you've done this, as I have. You look at a photo of yourself from the past, and it's just you in the photo and you are terribly cute, and you think, *My God, I wish I looked that cute now. I had no idea I was that cute. How could I not know?* You are by yourself in the photo, and the beauty and logic of your own body, your own look and limbs and length and width are just shining, and they don't mean anything but you, you, you. You are just you. There you are.

It's the context of the photo, that room or town or city. It's that culture. That's what made you ugly – or suspect that you might be. It was never you.

I've been fat all my life – other than those moments when my teenage starvation succeeded briefly to make me smaller. Even then, I was merely large, not fat. I am usually bigger than the other people in the photograph and comparison matters.

Girls are in constant comparison to one another. We are constantly compared, and we take up the task as taught.

I've been fat all my life. Another way to say this is that during my whole life, people have told me I was fat and treated me as damaged. Of course, I had no labels for my body when I was two or three years old. I had to be given the labels. 'If it's baby fat, why isn't it gone yet?' my father would ask my mother, accusingly, as though she should have an answer. He'd ask it while I stood there, blinking at them, at age two, then three. By four I knew to hide my too-fat legs when their gaze took on that scrutiny.

I remember him saying, 'Well, she gets those chubby knees from you.' My mother narrowed her eyes because, of course, she was the target of his insult, but the words ricocheted towards me as well. I was sitting on the floor playing with a toy in my nightgown and bathrobe, as they drank coffee on a weekend morning, and I pulled my clothes down to cover my terrible knees. I looked up to see my mother's knees, but they were already covered by her longer gown, though she was not fat. She had already removed her knees from view.

Very young, I knew it was important not to have chubby anything. It was important to both of my parents, and to others too. They'd look me up and down and cock their heads and say with a tone of pity laced with envy, 'She has such a pretty face.' I was failing a lot and succeeding a little. That's what I learned, and it was up to me to be better at – at what? I wasn't *doing* anything but existing in the body I'd been given. None of us asked why it was important to look a certain way as children. We just learned how it would prompt others to behave towards us and what we must do in penitence.

Mostly now, when I look at those photos of me as a very

small child, I see a child that was not particularly fat – rather, robust, bigger than most other kids my age. But if I'm alone in the photo, I just see beauty.

Maybe as adolescents we begin to question, but often, not even then. Especially if a teenage girl is winning at the game of appearance, she doesn't question, she just smiles and takes the pageant prize. She tries to look right because she can succeed at looking right. The slightest non-conformity, though – especially one that someone mentions more than once – can turn girl to rebel. The mercurial power to revolt is a righteous gift teenagers offer to the world. Vivacity and rebellion and, hopefully, the cleverness to survive and befriend their bodies through their non-conformity.

Teenagers question culture. It's their job. *Why* do I have to wear the skirt, the makeup, the headscarf, the bra, shave my legs, put on a coat, put on a bikini, cover my legs, cover my hair, cover my shoulders, cover my chest, cover my belly? Teenage girls are still, in the United States, fighting for the right to wear tank tops on a hot day, like boys do, because girl bodies are still seen as inciting male lust. So say the adults who should know better because they've lived longer and endured and committed more atrocities, but adults still need teens to question culture. We need rebellion.

Teenage girls also learn that there is power in their bodies. The power to attract and direct attention is not nothing. Teenage girls learn that boys and men hate this power and will remind them at every turn that men's power is greater and that they will punish, hurt, maim and kill women with impunity, and as they see fit.

For girls who bleed and ovulate, there is one more peril possible: pregnancy.

Let me take a moment to be very clear about this, because so few people in this culture understand the matter properly: sex does not cause pregnancy.

As a practising lesbian, none of the copious and amazing sex I have had during the past thirty years has put me in any danger of becoming pregnant. None of the casual or committed sex, boring or irritating sex, none of the sex in the car, on the kitchen table, on the bed or in the shower – no sex, ever, during those decades – has caused me to think I might be pregnant.

That's because sex doesn't cause pregnancy. Even doctors don't always understand this, and it seems like they should! They'll ask before an x-ray, are you sexually active? And then follow a positive response with, well, we'll just do this pregnancy test first . . .

This speaks volumes for how disrespected women's bodies are by the medical establishment and how little emphasis is placed on male responsibility for procreation. Indeed, if someone's trying to consider a man's familial responsibilities, the only question he's asked is whether he's married, not how many children he has or how often he's recently placed his sperm near a womb.

That would be the salient question. Where has he placed his sperm? There are so many places a man can eject his sperm that also put him at no risk of fatherhood. Down the shower drain means no pregnancy, into a tissue, into someone's mouth or someone's armpit, into the wind on a mountaintop or into the rolling surf. No chance of pregnancy. Sperm, near a womb, creates a chance for pregnancy. Not sex.

Women learn that pregnancy is a peril that we cannot fully control in a world where our bodies are thought to incite sex and sex is believed to cause pregnancy. Women are more likely to be raped than men, and more likely to be raped repeatedly. Men are almost always the rapists, and the type of rape men choose often places sperm near the womb. They know fully what the consequences are, and they do it anyway.

For many women, even those who have wanted and had children, the ability to control their fertility is a powerful strategy for opening the doors of their own life desires. Birth control or infertility – whether medically provoked or through menopause – will not make a woman un-rapeable, but it will allow her to avoid the choice (and manifold perils – social and medical) of abortion or pregnancy.

Menopause might be a more welcome and celebrated event for more women if it weren't also heralding the body's changes that render us invisible, unviable and unworthy of attention in a culture that already values everything about our humanity and contributions less if we're not seen as 'fuckable' by men.

I have been fat all my life. But there are different ways of being fat. I started out as a robust snake goddess and I'm ageing into the Venus of Willendorf. (Google those images if you're not familiar.) It took me a while to see all the nuances of fatness because I was fat in a privileged way and all people with privilege work hard not to see what they have. At least at first. I was too distracted by the challenge of being seen as fat to fully see my privilege as a teen and young adult. I had to be ingenious with fashion, where others just bought things off the rack. I had to be extra-diligent if I was going to be seen as just a regular participant at the gym, or in dating. How was I privileged? Remember the pretty face? This is a way of saying that part of my appearance was conforming.

Specifically, that part of my appearance was conforming to white supremacist, youth-focused, non-disabled, upper-class beauty standards.

Without overthinking, give a quick answer to these questions: Is it more acceptable for a woman to have a fat belly or fat thighs? Fat thighs or fat ankles? Fat back or fat boobs? Not all fat is seen equally. And above all, we are supposed to remain gender-conforming. Think about men. Fat is far more excusable on a man than a woman – unless he carries it in his boobs, or his hips and thighs. If it's a fat belly or back or a thick chest, he's more likely to be seen as a 'big guy', which is pretty good. If fat feminises his body – and particularly if he's short – his life chances are severely limited. Gender conformity is paramount.

By the time I was in my thirties, I owned my hotness and my privilege. Big butt, small waist, big boobs. I was what people like to call 'proportionate'. (Read: proportionate to dominant beauty standards.) Still too fat to be acceptable, still too wiggly, but yeah, I worked out and was strong and smart and cute and more impressive than most people in most ways. I had to be – just to be considered competent, dateable. Even still, most of the people I dated needed to be 'brought along' because I was the first fat babe they'd ever dated. So tedious, but I did the work of helping them realise that their bodies were also good bodies, because that's often the biggest barrier to loving other bodies: accepting our own.

One day, at my local nude resort, I was climbing into the hot tub, au naturel, with some other folks and I looked down at my own body and saw my belly just hanging there in a certain way. A roll had developed above my waistline but below my boobs. What the hell was that? I was forty-three years old. And on that day, I realised that body acceptance is not just something you do once. It's a thing you do again and again until you die because the body keeps changing and, in fact, ramps up its efforts around menopause. I wasn't disgusted with my body, but I felt suddenly self-conscious, aware of how I must look to others. I took a deep breath.

I was challenged again in my mid-forties when arthritis caused my yoga practice to become gentler; my walking and dancing and leaping became greatly curtailed. I didn't give up easily, though. My desire to keep doing with my body as I had always done created one injury after another. Now I walk with a limp. Wouldn't you think that a person with as much body awareness, who engages in critical analysis of body hierarchy and the relationship between self-love and political equity – wouldn't you think I'd have been able to avoid that level of self-harm? Apparently not. I was attached to my image of myself as capable in very specific ways. Devalued though my appearance was, I was attached to my own version of youth and beauty. Most of us are and it comes up in a variety of ways. I asked a friend recently if she'd been experiencing any troubling symptoms of perimenopause or menopause. We're both in our fifties. She quickly told me she wasn't. And wasn't going to. And didn't even want to talk about it. To her, that was for people who weren't fit and were somehow discontent with their lives and didn't take care of their health. She was just going to avoid troubling symptoms through magical thinking, it seemed to me. Or by denying the experience and avoiding discussions about it. I couldn't tell which.

I didn't bother to tell her that I've also not experienced many symptoms of menopause. Who knows why. Some brain fog, yes, but I've also recently been diagnosed with sleep apnoea, and now that I'm sleeping better, machine-aided, I'll see if the brain fog clears up. I had a 'night sweat' standing still in a cool museum one afternoon and that led me to understand that, wow, I haven't been having those, or hot flashes. It was like a fountain opened on the top of my head and suddenly sweat was pouring down my face and shoulders. These moments have been isolated, but who knows. We like to think we're in charge, but we're not. Literally, who knows what could happen next with my specific body?

Of course, a person's emotional state, cultural circumstances and overall sense of wellness influence physical symptoms. So far as I can tell, humans have little conscious control over how it all rolls together, and when the body hurts, it's going to be humbling. Maybe it's best to practise humility ahead of time.

Neoliberalism has all but squashed humility. If you perform well on a test, it's because you're a genius, not because you were trained for the task and the test was written for you. My mother used to say of any thin person we might be dining with, 'Well, just look at her. Obviously, she should be giving out the diet tips!' My teacher once commented on Spanish speakers being better at their own language if they happened to be Spanish rather than Mexican. 'Europeans just sound better,' he quipped. (Is this really neoliberal, or just racist? So many social phenomena are a combination.)

If you're fat or unemployed, the neoliberal ideology sees personal deficit. You should feel shame and work hard to repair your shortcomings. At no point is humility possible because interconnectedness is denied. Structural analysis is incompatible with personal responsibility.

Nowadays, the humblebrag supplants humility. 'I'm so humbled by this award.' It's an Orwellian doublespeak road to neoliberal-land. Actually, an award exalts the recipient. That's literally what it's designed to do. Feeling humbled happens when you don't get the award, but you keep doing a good job anyway. It happens when your front tooth gets knocked out, or you spill tomato soup down your whole shirt right before getting up to talk in front of a group. Humility is when you didn't make the right choice, but a lot of other people did and now you yearn to be better.

Seeing my belly rise and my skin sag humbles me, but it doesn't shame me. I remember what the practice of peace is for. Even though people will see me as less credible because of a fat, ageing, disabled body, I will do the work to rise into my vast and beautiful self again and again. When I can't do it for myself, I will do it for others. I will become a worthy participant in the great fabric of humanity because others need to see me do so in precisely this body. (I need to see your worthiness in your body as well. Please show me.)

Over the years, I've taught many retreats – healing, educational, restorative. Once, at a retreat where we were practising yoga and exploring the stories we carry in our bodies, a participant made a discovery. She began to question why she was so attached to her body not changing. Though she was slender and athletic, an injury caused her to see that she had been placing so much of her identity in the appearance of her body and how she didn't want it to change.

Athletes want to stay at pinnacle ability. Most women want to stay at pinnacle beauty, according to social standards, even though these may be conditions we've never really attained. Many women keep that one photograph, taken at the perfect angle, with amazing clothes and hair and makeup. It may look nothing like the person her friends and family love, but it's proof. She can say, 'I looked like that once!'

'Why should I want the body to stay stagnant?' my retreat participant said. I mean, if I want to do different things with my life, or have a baby, my body is going to change! Why is that a bad thing?

I had practised the acceptance of a certain body and thought that was enough. I didn't want it to change. Stagnation is what we seek. How do we admit that, and then see what it means? There is no current, no flow in stagnant water. It becomes stale, sluggish and dull from inaction. It becomes toxic to all who would attempt contact. I don't want anything about me to become stagnant – least not my appearance, the thing I share with others daily. I want an exchange of oxygen and life moving through my body as I interact with you, as I evolve into me.

This is one of the lessons of menopause, whether the transition, the ageing, influences us positively or negatively, or we don't notice physical changes at all. Don't stagnate. More importantly, refuse to stagnate at precisely the time when your culture tries hardest to eradicate you.

The culture wants to erase us as we age, and that's enough to make pain and hardship settle into the non-conforming body – no matter what we think we've handled in our heads. The body changes; menopause brings change. When Sophia Loren was asked, in her seventies, what she did to maintain her beauty, she said she didn't grunt and groan when moving. Things still hurt, but she didn't show the pain. There's wisdom in this response, if it's not taken too far. I hope that her calculation of how to respond to the challenges of ageing includes a deep inner peace.

We can choose how to respond to what the body feels, and experience the power of curating our appearance. And what more? Is it possible to show the pain without dwelling in it as our only home? It is indeed one experience of the ageing body. What else is there? What sensual pleasures and release into rest can be discovered in the ageing body? What pleasure in sexuality uncoupled from media stories of hotness and desirability? I want to know. Love is a practice. Self-love in a society that hates the female body (and browner women's bodies even more) is radical and necessary. I am grateful to Audre Lorde for showing us.

My body is an instrument that has already learned to sound in symphony with so many others. Love is the everyday practice of being at peace in the body, being in the company of others responsibly. Every experience wants to be heard and honoured, and I'll still be careful on which I shine a spotlight. Menopause is one more bit of sheet music to learn, one more way to practice love, justice and care.

Kimberly Dark (she/her) is a writer, sociologist and storyteller, working to reveal the architecture of everyday life so that we can reclaim our power as social creators. She's the author of four books, including *Fat, Pretty and Soon to be Old: A Makeover for Self and Society* and *Damaged Like Me: Essays on Love, Harm and Transformation*. Her essays, poetry and stories are widely published in academic and popular publications alike. She teaches for CSU Summer Arts and travels to offer keynotes, workshops and lectures internationally and online. Learn more and sign up for *The Hope Desk* newsletter at www.kimberlydark.com

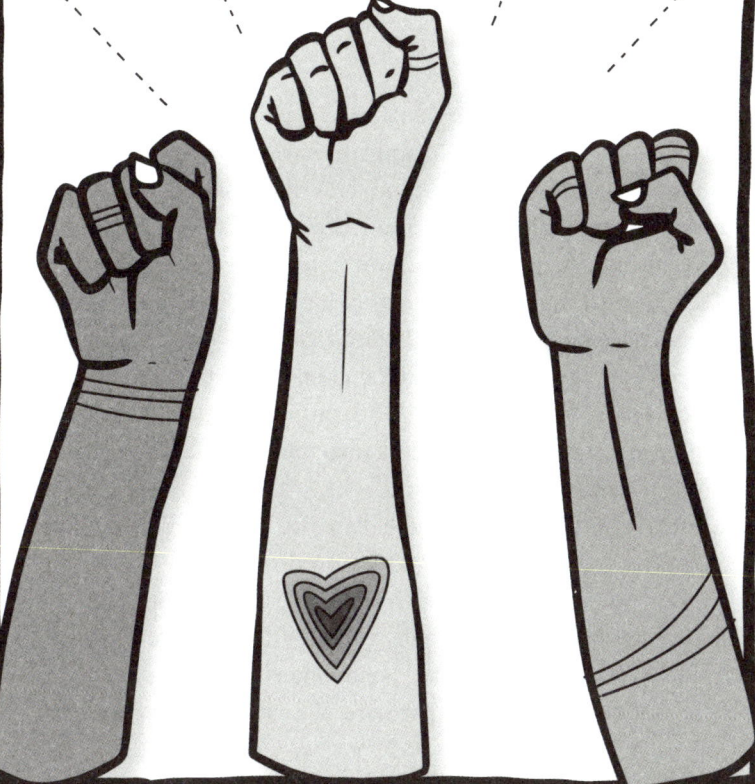

Sex and the Menopausal Vagina in the Suburbs

Susan Cole

'The good news is you don't have syphilis. The bad news is you're HIV-positive. Oh, and you have about seven years to live.' That's how I received my HIV diagnosis in 1999, from a balding, white immigration doctor, who eyed me with revulsion-tinged curiosity. (I'd moved to Louisiana from London to marry my second ex-husband. I've had three so far, collected like stamps.) I wasn't meant to still be alive. Yet here I am, going through the menopause almost twenty-five years later, back in the UK. With misinformation, stigma and judgement affecting women living with HIV still fucking up our lives as we get older.

Of course, the doctor who diagnosed me was wrong about my life expectancy. HIV had moved on by the late 1990s. HIV was no longer a death sentence, at least for people in rich countries. Today people with HIV on effective treatment can expect to live as long as anyone else. It's impossible to pass it on to our sexual partners. We can have children born free of HIV (I've had two before and two since my diagnosis – all HIV-negative). So, everything should be cool now, right? Actually, no. Particularly for menopausal women of colour living with HIV who face intersecting forms of stigma, discrimination and disadvantage.

I didn't expect to be alive to go through the menopause. I certainly didn't expect to be alive to go through the menopause twice, once because of chemotherapy. I've been told I should be grateful. Yet the narrative that women with HIV, particularly Black women, should be 'grateful' for merely being alive is sometimes used as an oppressive, patriarchal tool to silence us. So we don't challenge the abuse and disrespect we regularly experience. So our expectations are decimated and substandard healthcare seems appropriate. So our self-worth is crushed by a tsunami of societal stigma that drowns out our warning inner voice.

Women living with HIV are told we should be grateful if a man stays with us. That he is the glorious hero, brave for being in a relationship with a sullied woman with HIV. This narrative can shackle us, keeping us in abusive relationships. Often abusers tell us 'no other man will want you now', that we are unworthy of love. Throw in being classified as 'menopausal' and therefore supposedly past our prime and value in society, our self-esteem can be further decimated. Should I therefore go silent into that good night of cowed matronly oblivion? Fuck that. I choose shameless meteor-like blazing.

But first, let's go back to menopause number one: the surprise, chemotherapy-induced version. Who knew chemotherapy could bring on an early menopause? Certainly not me. It was in January 2012 when I first felt a lump in my breast. I was 'lucky' to have been referred for a mammogram, ultrasound and even a biopsy – yet the doctors dismissed the results as only showing 'dense breasts' and 'cysts'. I didn't know then that Black women are more likely to be diagnosed late with cancer and more likely to die than white women. It was actually having HIV that saved my life. Six months after the 'cysty dense breasts' misdiagnosis, I saw my fabulous HIV consultant Dr Charlotte Cohen, who insisted I go back for more tests, as I'd mentioned to her I'd developed a rash on my breasts. This time the cancer was found. Triple-negative breast cancer. One of the most aggressive types. With the worst outcomes. Disproportionately affecting Black women. Perceived death sentence number two – this time with four children, two under the age of ten.

When my breast cancer was *finally* diagnosed, the tumour was 5 cm across and down. Fortunately, not spread anywhere else, but so big that chemotherapy was essential. I don't recall the elderly, bloated oncologist telling me that a possible outcome would be an early, more intense menopause, or anything else I should expect. What I do recall vividly is him having a perverse interest in my HIV status. How did I get it? What was I to do to not pass it on to my husband? Him scrawling 'HIV positive', circled in red pen on a form. Women with HIV are most likely to experience stigma in healthcare settings like this, when we are at our most vulnerable, and it can be difficult to challenge it. I didn't at the time, nor did I ask the questions I wanted. I was blindsided by his ignorance and the stigma, simultaneously traumatised by my cancer diagnosis. I did complain later and changed hospitals. But I missed the vital opportunity to get prepared for what was coming. Including the menopause.

I can't lie. Chemotherapy is shit. I expected the possibility of losing my hair and feeling a little queasy. Not the onslaught of toxic, cancer-killing chemicals surging through the rest of my body, sledgehammering healthy cells in their rampage. Not that the chemotherapy would attack my ovaries and start the menopause. So, on top of the projectile vomiting, nerve burning, hair obliteration and plot-twist anaphylaxis, I was also hot flushing, memory losing and mood swinging with such intensity I didn't think I would survive. No one told me that I could have an early menopause because of chemotherapy. Nor that the symptoms of a chemo-induced menopause would likely be more severe. I assumed symptoms were just part of the slasher-horror show of chemo, but when my periods stopped, I suspected it could be the menopause.

I was eventually told it was likely I was experiencing early menopause because of chemotherapy, and likely it would be permanent. I was crushed. Not because I couldn't have more children, but it felt like cancer had permanently changed me. The chemotherapy, with radiotherapy and surgery, appeared to have worked (the cancer has not come back, for now at least), but I was altered. I was left with permanent nerve damage, a constant twist of terror in my stomach that the cancer would return, and chemically shrivelled ovaries. I felt less of a woman. This coincided with my husband leaving and a hellish, traumatic divorce.

When your life is imploding as you go through the menopause, with a dash of HIV thrown in, it can be hard to pinpoint what's causing the symptoms. Brain fog so all-encompassingly thick it clouds your memory to the extent you repeat yourself? That's intense stress, right? Or a chemotherapy effect? Or having to swap your HIV meds because of chemo? Or all, or some, or something else, something more serious, cancer spread to the brain? I stumbled hairless through the next few months, drowning in trauma and confusion. I didn't have the time to investigate symptoms of the menopause. All I knew about was hot flushes. I didn't know menopause could cause brain fog. And no one told me. I crumpled silently.

And then, as suddenly as it arrived, the menopause was gone. My ovaries were simply in a Sleeping Beauty slumber, cursed but not killed by the nefarious spinning wheel of chemotherapy. Just when I was beginning to celebrate no longer having periods, they were back in bloody vengeance. All symptoms of the menopause just dissipated – no more mood swings and hot flushes and memory loss. But yet again, no explanation from my general practitioner (or GP in the UK); it was up to me to try to figure it out. I read that for the majority of women who had a chemo-induced menopause it would likely be temporary. And that the average age for the *real* menopause was fifty-one. So, it would be about eight years until I had the menopause again, right? Wrong, three years later the menopause came crashing into my life again.

Women with HIV *may* have the menopause earlier and *may* experience worse symptoms. That, apparently, is the scientifically correct thing to say, as some studies indicate that's the case while others do not. But seriously, what the fuck does that actually mean to a woman living with HIV whose life is being brutally ravaged by what may or may not be menopause symptoms? And *may* or *may not* be happening earlier than other women? And what does it mean to many doctors who seem to be eager to find a simple diagnostic box to tick regarding a set of symptoms within the allocated five minutes, before moving on to the next patient, then the next, then the next?

Five minutes is often all we get with our GP. The doctor who is meant to diagnose everything as efficiently as possible. That's if we actually manage to see one in the first place. It can be a quest of Herculean magnitude to bypass the hawk-eyed receptionist gatekeeper who decides if you're worthy to speak to a doctor or not.

I say 'speak to', not see. You see, the vast majority of 'appointments' since Covid are terse phone calls. Not the best for trying to explain that you're sweating, and weeping, and pissing, and burning, and aching, and forgetting, and ballooning, and SCREAMING. Screaming as your health and libido and sense of self unravel. Yet you have to keep going, as you have no choice because everyone relies on you. That's how it can feel for some of us women going through the menopause. But it can be somewhat of a challenge to articulate that in a five-minute telephone dialogue with a locum GP you've never spoken to before.

Chances are, *if* we do get to see a GP, they'll tell us blithely it's an 'HIV issue' and refer us back to our HIV doctor. And then the endless ping-ponging begins. From the GP to the HIV doctor, back to the GP, back to the HIV doctor. Sometimes, if we do have another health condition (and so many of us women with HIV do), then that specialist (in my case a urologist) gets added into this perverse human pass the parcel.

I suppose if I had to pick one menopause symptom to be my 'thing', it would be repeat urinary tract infections (UTIs). Not the sanitised version that a nice fresh glass of cranberry juice allegedly magics away. But the version in which pissing is passing razors lacerating your vagina as you eject clots of blood and pus, with pain so intense you think you'll throw up and pass out. The version in which the infection snakes up your ureter and savages your kidneys so now you are throwing up and burning up and in hospital pumped with intravenous antibiotics. That version.

Many women with HIV going through the menopause have spoken to me about repeat UTIs, and how little is done to help them. I'm on daily antibiotics to keep them at bay, but it only seems to take missing a dose, or actually just looking at a man, and an infection comes surging back.

Yes, that would be sex. Women with HIV have sex. Menopausal women with HIV have sex. That seems to make some people upset – the thought of women, stigmatised both for having HIV *and* no longer being fertile. Patriarchy objectifies women to the extent that our value is often perceived to come from fertility and youth. So, if we're menopausal yet still wanting to have sex, we're a grotesque aberration. Add in having what is primarily a sexually transmitted virus, regardless of whether we can transmit HIV or not, we're an abomination.

Women with HIV who speak about our need for sexual pleasure may face slut-shaming abuse. That was certainly my experience when I wrote for the HIV magazine *Positive Nation* and had a regular column called 'Sex and the Suburbs' in the 2000s, discussing navigating relationships and sex as a woman living shamelessly with HIV. I would get hate mail, primarily from some embittered white gay men, who accused me of lying – I couldn't possibly be having fun and sex; that was either not their experience or, if it was, it was exclusively their thing! In fact, HIV was their thing; women shouldn't be muscling into the HIV narrative with swearing and sex and fun!

The abuse ramped up when I was photographed naked for

the cover of the magazine – seven months pregnant lying on sheepskin in five-inch Gucci heels. ('Sensual' was how the singer Sam Smith described it recently, after seeing it for a BBC podcast series on HIV we were both in.) I didn't do it for attention (although I love attention, something else women are hated for) but to show, with the feature on pregnancy I wrote, that women with HIV could have children born free of HIV. That apparently made them feel sick, made them take the time to write letters dripping with venom about how, when I die of AIDS, my children will be so ashamed of me. Well, you know what, I'm still here and my children are proud of me. And along with the hate letters, there were actually more with love, including from a pregnant woman with HIV who wrote to say she was being coerced into having a termination by her doctor – he argued women with HIV couldn't have children. My article and photo showed her he was wrong and she went on to have her baby, born without HIV. Who knew you could do some good from being an attention-seeking slut?

And I continue to write and talk about sex, including through the menopause. But that seems to make some people uncomfortable. Maybe that's why discussions on menopause seem to focus on the safer symptoms – hot flushes and a spot of comedic 'menopause brain'. Not symptoms relating to our menopausal vaginas. Not loss of libido, or painful sex, or dry vaginas, or genital itching, or UTIs or vaginal atrophy. And too often we're shamed into silence. And if we do gather the courage to speak to a doctor, many of us won't get the help we need.

The situation is worse for women with HIV. The PRIME Study, one of the largest studies globally on HIV and menopause, led by feminist HIV consultant Dr Shema Tariq at

University College London (UCL), found that women in England living with HIV aged between forty-five and sixty were more likely to report a range of sexual problems than women without HIV in the same age group.[1] Women with HIV were also more likely to report an increase in sexual problems during the menopause; less than 5 per cent reported taking vaginal oestrogen, which can help some of the vaginal symptoms (such as dryness) of menopause. I spoke to Dr Tariq about these findings, who said: 'Ageism and sexism combine to silence discussions about older women's sex lives. Then of course you have racism, and the neglect of sexual pleasure as an important part of our [brown and Black] female experience. And, finally, HIV is added to the mix. Historically, discourse about HIV and sex is centred upon risk [preventing HIV], rather than pleasure. My work is focused on viewing sex through an intersectional lens, and empowering women with HIV through information, so they can enjoy the sex they want, regardless of their age.'

The PRIME Study also highlighted the shocking racial inequity affecting Black women with HIV going through the menopause in England. In this study, Black African women were more likely to have a university education than white women, but more likely to live in poverty. They were also more likely to report psychological distress but less likely to be diagnosed with depression, so therefore not getting the help they need.

Surprising? Hell no, not to Black women, at least. We know we've been experiencing health inequalities for generations, across medical conditions, fuelled by structural racism. Just in the UK we're four times more likely than white women to die in childbirth,[2] more likely to be diagnosed late with cancer and therefore die from the disease.[3] And for those of us who think our economic privilege may prevent it, think again. You don't get more economically privileged than Serena Williams, yet she nearly died giving birth to her daughter, suffering from a pulmonary embolism and a ruptured C-section after her concerns were initially dismissed.

They try to put the blame on us, say we're 'hard to reach' and use terms like 'hesitant' and 'untrusting'. Of course, some of us are going to be fucking untrusting if we've faced doctors treating us with disregard and disrespect and disbelief. And if we do say our treatment is because of racism, we're gaslit by the media and politicians – we're told we have chips on our shoulders or are playing the race card. That *they* are the real victims of our 'wokery'.

These racial health inequities absolutely apply to menopause. A review of twenty-five years of research on menopause in the USA, the SWAN Study, found that Black women had worse menopause symptoms but were less likely to receive medical help. We were more likely than white women to experience symptoms like depression, sleep disturbances and hot flushes – but at the same time less likely to get medical and mental health support and receive hormone therapy.

I know hormone replacement therapy, also known as HRT, may not be for everyone (for instance, for women like me who've had breast cancer); however, if it's being denied to us even though it can make our life and health better, there's something seriously fucked up going on there.

There's a misconception that HRT is a short-term fix for some symptoms of the menopause, like hot flushes, and once you're through the menopause, your health just magically repairs. The reality is very different. The hormone oestrogen has a protective effect against inflammation, which is linked to many serious health conditions. It's why before the menopause, women don't have high rates of heart disease, stroke and Alzheimer's disease. I spoke to Dr Nneka Nwokolo, a sexual health consultant with extensive expertise on the menopause, about this. She said: 'The question is, when your oestrogen levels go down, what happens to rates of heart disease? Well, we know they go up. Women stop being protected and their rate of heart disease goes up as high as, and sometimes higher than, in men. Studies have shown that menopause increases the risk of comorbidities above that just associated with ageing. We know that if you give HRT within a ten-year window of becoming menopausal, rates of heart disease remain low. Rates of osteoporosis remain low. Rates of Alzheimer's disease remain low.'

She stressed that this was important for women with HIV, who already have higher rates of inflammation, even when we're on effective treatment. This may be linked to still having reservoirs of HIV in our bodies, as well as to our lifestyles, but often also because of the increased stress many of us experience throughout our lives. And we know now that HRT can be helpful for women with HIV, to protect us from these diseases we are already disproportionately affected by. Yet we're less likely to be prescribed it by doctors.

I've been running peer-led discussion workshops, primarily for Black women with HIV going through the menopause, and the same stories keep coming up. Suffering harrowing symptoms, but the doctor isn't interested. Asking about HRT but being told it's not appropriate for them. Suffering in silence as they simultaneously grapple with poor housing, stigma, poverty, violence, a hostile immigration system, racism. Drowning in responsibilities and overwork. 'Why bother saying anything when no one is going to do anything about it?' is a frequent refrain.

Well, you know what? I'm going to fucking bother. This oppressive patriarchal society would like us to be silenced, cowed by abuse and shame. Grateful for crumbs of inadequate care. But they've got us wrong. One thing we women with HIV who've managed to get to menopause possess is resilience. We've been through so much shit but we're still here. We are not the passive, voiceless victims they would like to believe us to be.

Knowledge is one of the most empowering weapons we have. It's important to know our own bodies. Know our rights so we can challenge poor healthcare and instead get the gold standard of care we deserve. Know about the options to maximise our health, so we can make informed decisions about what works best for us as individuals. Use our collective voices and talents to lead the fight against the system and bring about meaningful change for us all.

But one of the most important things we can do is cast off the shroud of shame and guilt that weighs down so many women with HIV. And that's what I'm doing. I choose shameless self-love, including for my menopausal, HIV-positive vagina.

Susan Cole (she/her) is an international public speaker, broadcaster, writer, activist, and health equity changemaker. Starting her cross sector career as a research psychologist, with time in the corporate arena, she moved on to have over two decades of leadership in the HIV and sexual health sector, spearheading innovative initiatives with national and global impact, particularly for women and people of colour. She is a London-based, three-times-divorced intersectional feminist and mother of four. Find out more at SusanColeHaley.com

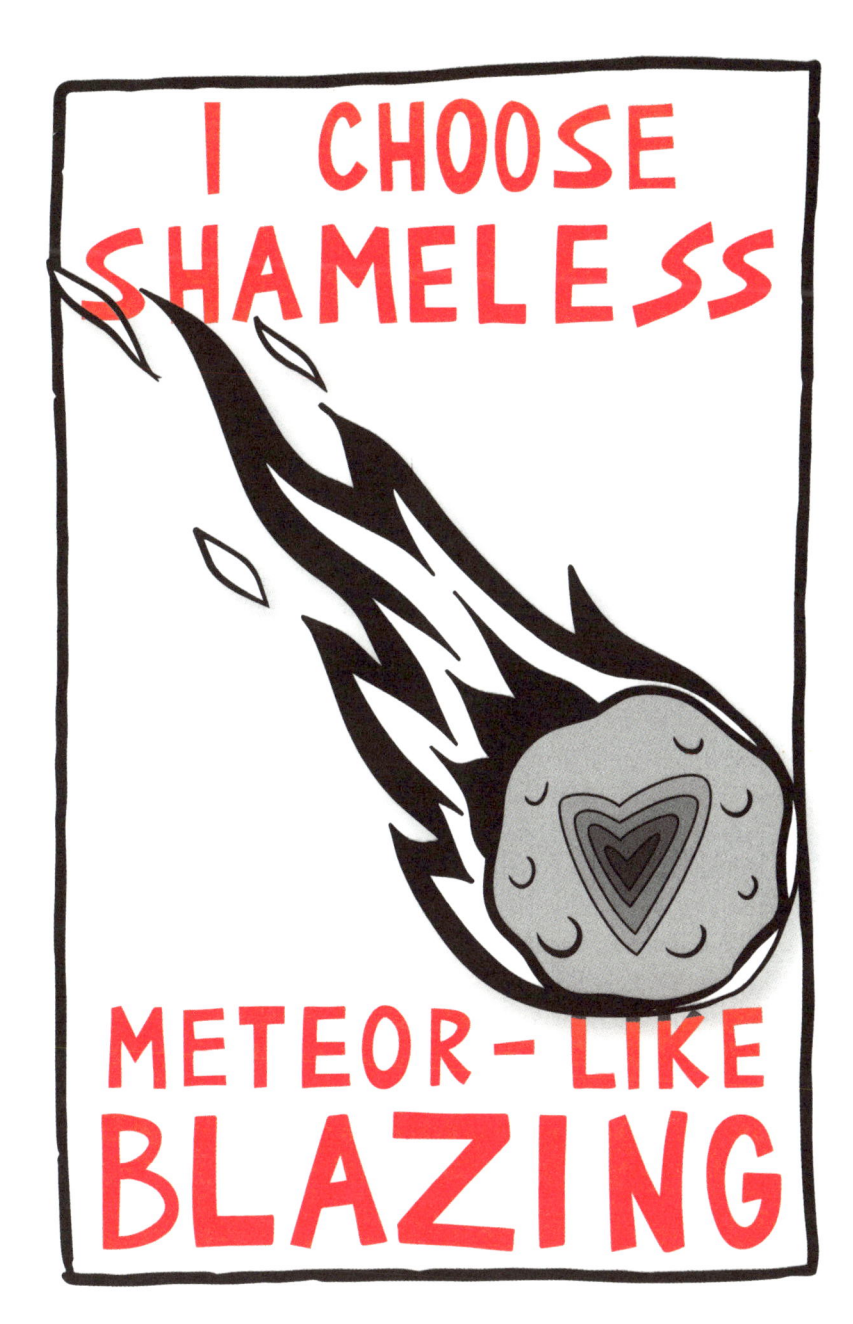

I CHOOSE SHAMELESS METEOR-LIKE BLAZING

Where Do I End? Wherever I Begin

Una Mullally

In the summer of 2015, I was locked in a hospital bathroom rationing the depleting tissue left in the dispenser, knowing there was never going to be enough to dry my tears. I was crying in that desperate, heaving way, the kind of upset for which there's little comfort and certainly no consolation. You know the type of bawling I'm talking about. It's the distraught kind, the unravelling kind, the kind that when you catch your reflection in the smudged mirror of wherever you've barricaded yourself into, you're shocked by the extremity of what the weeping session has revealed on your face. Well, *I* was, anyway, seeing my beetroot head, wet cheeks, hair sticking to my forehead, my tears the adhesive. With each passing knock on the door, I blurted 'busy' or 'out in a minute', in that octave-too-high pretence of stability. When my tear ducts had wrung empty, I tried to get my shit together, splashing cold water on my face, dabbing my eyes with my t-shirt in the towel-less cubicle, breathing deep air in juddering sighs.

This standoff against myself was occurring in the aftermath of a signature, my own name written on a consent form that was placed in front of me with all the casualness of a package-delivery confirmation, or a new phone contract. I had attended an appointment hoping for a positive outcome to my predicament, but during the conversation with the gynaecologist surgeon, that hope was rapidly revealed to be a delusion. What I wanted was for one of my ovaries to be saved. What I got was a consent form for a hysterectomy and an ovariectomy of both ovaries. Within a couple of weeks, both my womb and ovaries would be gone.

I was thirty-two years old, and this wasn't even the worst thing going on in my life. I had stage three colorectal cancer, had undergone six weeks of daily radiation therapy, six weeks of constant chemotherapy, and was on the precipice of major surgery to remove a tumour, lymph nodes and multiple other bits and pieces. And then this.

The potential impact of cancer treatment on my fertility was drip-fed to me by doctors, surgeons and nurses. Initially, after my staging determined the cancer wasn't terminal and a treatment plan could be devised, I was asked to think about freezing my eggs, while simultaneously told that such a procedure needed to happen as quickly as possible to prevent it from delaying cancer treatment. I gave that option a few hours' thought, and decided against it. I didn't realise that my next period would be my last. There was a risk, I was told, of infertility due to the radiation. That did indeed happen. My uterus was battered by the treatment and needed to go. Secondary cancers were a worry. The radiation had such an impact that within a couple of years I would fracture my lower back in two places, and my pain receptors were so fried that these injuries weren't revealed by me reporting pain, but by check-up x-rays.

I pictured my irradiated womb like a glowing lava lamp at the base of my torso, humming its neon haze. I thought of my ovaries struggling to survive, imagining a cartoonish skit as they attempted to stay out of harm's way, little Indiana Jones globs, pinning themselves back on a dizzying ledge, with pebbles crumbling into the chasm below.

I was already experiencing menopausal symptoms – hot flashes, insomnia, mood swings, depression, incandescent rage, night sweats – but there was so much other stuff going on with and in my body and mind that segmenting these symptoms and connecting them to menopause specifically felt impossible.

I hadn't even yet heard the terms 'surgical menopause' or 'radical menopause' – the experience of entering into menopause overnight due to the surgical removal of one's uterus and ovaries. Radical menopause felt appropriate as a name for what was happening. I was too consumed by the edge of my own mortality to properly conceptualise, or even give the necessary credence to, the hormonal depletion, the bedrock of my reproductivity crumbling, the extraction of the parts that made me biologically female. When that reality met me, my signature blurring in my tear-filling eyeballs as I wrote my name on the consent form, I felt the end of something I had never dedicated much thought to: the intersection of my personal fertility and my individual femaleness. Where does a woman begin, and where does one end? Where did I begin, if I was a woman? And what was I ending? Or was this even any of that?

Menopause is seen as synonymous with ageing. But I was young. I had never thought about the medical reality of what happens later in life, and if I had, menopause was to be filed on the long finger, like pensions and retirement plans, neither of which I had (and still don't).

As my body was engaged in its own battle, or whatever other unhelpful cancer metaphor I could conjure, my country, Ireland, was drawing new battle lines around the bodies of women. As I recovered, almost miraculously, from cancer – albeit with huge long-lasting complications – Ireland was gripped by the reproductive rights movement and the drive to hold a referendum campaign to repeal the Eighth Amendment, our constitutional ban on abortion. I was still a woman, I was still fighting this battle, but its constitutional trenches were no longer my own bodily ones.

I found myself at marches where the old chants rang through Dublin's streets: 'Get your rosaries off our ovaries.' I would hear this chant, and absentmindedly think: 'I don't have ovaries, though.' The common biological and physiological ground I shared with my sisters was now absent within me. A common cliché during that campaign was to say that no woman in Ireland of childbearing age had voted for the Eighth Amendment. The referendum that introduced the amendment into the Irish constitution happened in 1983, the year I was born. Thirty-five years later, we would vote to remove it.

Now that I was a woman 'of childbearing age' without the anatomical equipment to bear those hypothetical children, I began to question the fundamentals of my gender. What made me female? Biologically, physically, socially, politically? I am a dyke, and for my whole life, I have experienced cis, straight women not seeing me as fully female. While characteristics of my biological sex had been removed surgically, in conversations with cis, straight women, my sexuality often appeared to be collapsed into a version of gender they did not relate to, and therefore could not see. Lesbians did not appear to be women *like them*.

During the abortion referendum, discussions about another referendum campaign, the Irish referendum on marriage equality in 2015, were frequent. It was referenced all the time. One of the things that cis, straight women who were more engaged in the abortion referendum than they had been in the marriage-equality referendum would say to me was: 'This must have been what it was like for you in 2015,' as though I wasn't also fighting for abortion rights, as though I wasn't a woman *like them* because I'm a lesbian, as though the emotional impact of 2015's referendum hit my identity hard, and yet I couldn't possibly feel the same – or worse! – in 2018's referendum. I would answer: yes, it was hard in 2015, and it's also hard now, because I am also a woman fighting for my bodily autonomy, as I am a lesbian who fought for her relationship recognition. In those moments, I realised how lesbians were perceived as outside womanhood and femaleness by so many cis, straight women, while I was also hurting over this new inner trauma I had experienced through surgery. I wondered what to do with this affront, while also feeling that in my own particular case, they were correct: I didn't have a womb to fight for (not that they knew that).

What's in a womb, I wondered? What does it really mean? What is the absence of ovaries really about? What does the end of reproductive capacity – or even prowess – signal for one's gender? What are bodily autonomy and reproductive rights when the parts of my body the constitution was obsessed with weren't personally relevant to me any more?

How do we continue to be women when the markers of our biology deplete or are removed? Why did it feel no one spoke about this beyond diffuse and opaque conversations about ageing? Where would I be categorised within the colonialist transphobic branch of feminism that had taken hold in Britain that appeared hell-bent on deciding what the borders of gender were with the kind of stance that asserted itself as always the officers in the mess, drawing lines on maps, and never the stance of those walking over those borders in the dead of night with belongings in supermarket bags? I was a woman, self-declared, decreed so at birth, never assuming another gender, yet some of the 'characteristics' of my womanhood were now gone. I began to wonder whether the other non-anatomical characteristics were ever really mine at all.

This existential gender spin was underpinned by societal silence around menopause. I knew why I had heard the term 'menopause' or 'menopausal' more frequently as a punchline than something to be discussed in genuine conversation, because menopause is correlated with ageing, and in my culture, older women are to be shoved aside, pitied, rendered useless, made invisible, de-centred from culture, ignored, joked about, reduced to clichés about grannies.

Clearly the answers I was looking for would not emerge from the colonialist horror imposed on Ireland, nor the now-fading theocracy which came after, and certainly not the reigning capitalism that leaped to the fore atop the ruins – the foundations still there – of that colonialism and that theocracy. I would have to look further, for new maps, for new relationships to gender, and for new feminisms. Angela Davis wrote in *Freedom Is a Constant Struggle: Ferguson, Palestine, and the Foundations of a Movement*:

Feminism involves so much more than gender equality and it involves so much more than gender. Feminism must involve consciousness of capitalism (I mean the feminism that I relate to, and there are multiple feminisms, right). So it has to involve a consciousness of capitalism and racism and colonialism and post-colonialities, and ability and more genders than we can even imagine and more sexualities than we ever thought we could name.

I felt that, big time.

And then, an email. Would I participate in an event about menopause in Dublin? The event was to be called Konenki, drawing not from white 'Western' thought around menopause, but from Japanese culture. In this context, menopause was seen as a period of liberation, not just from the risk of pregnancy, but also from the oppression of how society viewed womanhood itself.

I began to turn menopause on its head. If menopause – and ageing – was invisible, and therefore colluded in making women invisible, then what could happen in the darkness of invisibility? I thought of two other aspects of Japanese philosophy: of pottery and architecture. The first, kintsugi, the practice of repairing broken pottery, has found its way into broader global culture. Its underpinning sentiment – that there is beauty in brokenness, and that it is what's flawed that gives character – has been trivialised and Insta-flattened, but it is still wonderful. The second, I drew from Jun'ichirō Tanizaki's *In Praise of Shadows*, the seminal essay on Japanese aesthetics. 'Were it not for shadows,' Tanizaki wrote, 'there would be no beauty.' He wrote, 'If light is scarce then light is scarce; we will immerse ourselves in the darkness and there discover its own particular beauty.' It became obvious to me that, given such philosophy across aesthetics, of course menopause was treated differently in a culture that imagined beauty in such a specific way.

I am a fan of shadows, of absence, of the space between, of the underground and of the darkness. I am a fan of the hollow where nothing exists but possibility, murkiness, ambiguity, because that means uncertainty, and uncertainty means experimentation, and experimentation means potential, and potential means discovery. The unknown is where excitement and interesting things breed and emerge. We cannot be surprised by what we already know.

In my new menopausal state, I was the unknown. If my womb and ovaries were gone, invisible, what could their absence be filled with but an escape hatch from the tyranny of expectations, insults, pressures, attacks and oppressions meted out to women as punishment for having those biological attributes in the first place?

My society had formed my womanhood, with its gendered violence, and gender pay gaps, and catcalling, and constitutional inequality, and exclusion from medical research. That wasn't me. That was the scaffolding of discrimination that hemmed in the architecture of my personhood. Now my body had undergone a renovation. I realised that the anchors of biology were very loose indeed when it came to the broader interpretation of womanhood, femaleness and femininity. The things that made me a woman in the strict terms my society dictated were gone. And without them, I was strangely free. I was in the space between. I was unwomaned, as 'woman' is bluntly interpreted. Menopause, specifically surgical menopause, had gifted me ambiguity amid its trauma. Femaleness, like maleness, like all strict categories, was just that: a category. Its experience was taught by external forces. In the shadows, I searched.

In this search, I have repeatedly and intentionally unmoored myself. I never related to the female gender as it was performed in my society. I rejected the conservative markers of femininity, the conversations about female bodies, the male-gaze beauty standards, the expected way to dress and to act. I was never interested in the consumer behaviour of womanhood as capitalism. I didn't even engage in the endless chatter about periods because I never struggled with mine, and now they were over. I didn't care for the 'men are trash' discourse or the recycled second-wave gender-war discourse, because I didn't date men. I didn't fume about male bosses, because when I started out in journalism, my bosses were women, and then I became self-employed and I was my own boss. I didn't have the straight, cis, feminist lens that confused patriarchy with men. I wanted to confront systems, not individuals. If womanhood was all these things, it did not pertain to me. And then menopause removed me even further from this centralised category of 'woman', and especially of 'woman in her thirties'. What a gift. Had I not entered menopause so early, I would have had to wait for this gift, and by then, it would have been tied up in ageing, a whole other shitshow societies expect us to wade through because age segregation is so profound everywhere.

On the shadowy map of my new uncharted womanhood, I began to draw new islands. 'More genders than we can even imagine,' Davis wrote. More bodies. More versions. More interpretations. More declarations. Where does a woman end?

Where should she begin? Everywhere and nowhere, at sea and on land, underground and in the sky, in deep space, and in the recesses of one's tripping mind.

The shore of my womanhood was being eroded, and I was grateful for it. New dunes formed as new winds blew. New tides washed up with a new ebb and flow. I became myself, unrestricted from the markers that told me who I was, biologically, physically, socially, politically. I am the space between. I am not the formation of external factors. I am a new thing, a transforming thing, a metamorphosing thing, a dangerous thing because this thing is not set, it is not to be categorised, it is not to be labelled. I am a liberated thing within my own consciousness, a free radical, an untangled strand ripped from the tapestry of expectations.

Menopause is not a trap, it is not a slipway into irrelevance, it is not a cliff edge, it is not a cage, it is not a curse, it is not a burden. It is a gift, floating out beyond, a thing that can land at any time. Grab it with both fists. And then raise those fists, in defiance, in freedom.

Una Mullally (she/her) is a writer from Dublin, Ireland. As a journalist she writes columns and articles for newspapers, including weekly for the *Irish Times*, and occasionally for the *Guardian*. Her articles have also appeared in *Granta*, the *New York Times* and elsewhere. As an author she writes books such as *In the Name of Love* (2014), an oral history of the marriage-equality movement in Ireland, and the anthology *Repeal the 8th* (2018), which she edited. As a poet she writes poems, which she and others have performed in various places and at various times when and where poems are called for. As a screenwriter she co-writes films and TV with Sarah Francis. There are other things she does too, most of which relate to organising or contributing to things with a view to feeling alive.

GRAB IT WITH **BOTH FISTS** + RAISE THOSE FISTS IN FREEDOM

My Mother, the Menopause and Me

Nana Darkoa Sekyiamah

'I DON'T REMEMBER': INSIGHTS FROM MY MOTHER ON PREPARING FOR THE MENOPAUSE

I recently interviewed my mum about her experience of the menopause. It was the first time I recall ever sitting with her and talking openly and honestly about our bodies and the many transitions that come with age. I told her that I had heard that daughters tend to follow the menopause patterns of our mothers, and so I wanted to know what her journey through this life stage had been like. She started off by saying, 'When you menstruate early, your menopause also starts early.' I don't know if this is a medical fact, but it resonates with me.

My own period came like a red shock from the blue. I was twelve and had just started attending a Catholic boarding school in Accra, Ghana. Our school uniform was a white dress with blue bands across the collar and arms, and around the base of the skirt. The sack-like outfit was pulled together by a black belt whose width had to be a maximum of one inch. At assembly or simply walking around the school, you could be pulled over at random by a nun, teacher or senior prefect, who would whip out a tape measure to check if your belt was the regulation width. The only other part of our uniform was a navy-blue cardigan, which really came in handy when Auntie Flo appeared from nowhere. Oftentimes we would only realise we had had our periods when we stood up to find the seat of our pristine white school uniform stained a scarlet red. Out would come the blue cardigan, tied quickly around one's waist. But that too was against school rules: one was to wear their cardigan, not wrap it around one's waist. Our male French teacher in particular would demand that any girl he saw wearing a cardigan in a non-compliant fashion take it off immediately. She would then have to bashfully say, 'Please, sir: I have my period, and I've soiled my dress.' I was one of a few girls often caught in that situation.

From the moment my period started, she's been a source of shame and embarrassment: heavy, red and furious. In my early twenties I somewhat successfully controlled her by going on the combined contraceptive pill, sometimes taking it without a break because my periods were a major inconvenience. It felt freeing to be able to decide, 'This month I am not going to bleed.' That sense of liberation was cut short in my late twenties when my doctor took me off that medication because I had borderline high blood pressure. The progesterone-only pill that I was prescribed as an alternative made me break out in tiny pimples all over my back. I stopped taking it.

In my thirties I had an intrauterine device (IUD) installed because I had heard that it would stop my period, but I bled even more than I had ever done before. I once bled for thirty days non-stop. My gynaecologist assured me that everything was fine and that it could take up to six months for my body to adjust, and for the periods to stop. In my fifth month I went to a sexual health clinic for a routine STD test. I was handed a self-testing kit, which included a swab that I was instructed to insert high into my vagina, turn around a few times and then place in a sealed bag. When I pulled the swab out, I felt a sharp, searing pain and looked down to discover my IUD dangling at the end of the cotton bud. That was when I gave up on trying to use contraceptives to control my period.

I once read in a women's magazine that we should think of periods like seasons (in the West). Winter was like being on your period: a time to stay indoors, be comfy and drink warming soups. The writer urged the reader to take things easy, avoid scheduling key meetings and take time to nest. Ideologically, it made all the sense in the world to me, but – alas – the capitalist world we live in doesn't operate that way. Although it would be an intuitive way to operate, life doesn't pause around our biological clocks.

At the age of forty-two, I adopted my baby girl. 'That's it,' I thought. 'I don't need my periods any more.' I no longer felt the urge to try for biological children, as my daughter was already more perfect than any I could have genetically created. Three years later, my body got the message and I went three months without any sign of the red that had plagued most of my life. I went back to visit my gynaecologist, who ran a pregnancy test, confirmed that I didn't have a baby baking in my womb, and then ran some hormone tests. 'You have high levels of the hormones associated with the menopause. You're in the perimenopause stage.' I received this news with excitement. No more periods! No more fear of staining white sheets! No more mood swings! Alas: a month or so later, my period resumed, as heavy as ever before.

Knowing that I have firmly begun my journey towards the menopause, I have decided to be more proactive in seeking insights into what this new phase might mean for me. Interviewing my seventy-six-year-old mum about her own experience was really helpful in making me feel prepared for this transition, and gave me much insight into what else I could proactively do to sail through the menopause and all life transitions with aplomb. Right at the end of our interview, I asked her the one question every good interviewer knows to ask:

'Is there anything else you would like to share?'

'Yes,' she responded. 'Has your menopause started?'

'Yes, don't you remember? I told you that the doctor said I was perimenopausal.'

'No,' she retorted. 'I don't remember. That's one of the signs of the menopause.'

We both burst out laughing because she had just told me about one of her strategies for dealing with menopausal forgetfulness, something she had started to experience in her fifties. She would often walk from the kitchen to her bedroom to pick something up. Often forgetting upon arrival, she took to sitting on her bed until she remembered. She also told me about a time when she spent ages looking for her glasses, finally found them and put them on top of the spectacles she was already wearing. That's my mum: humorous and pragmatic. She shared with me that she had prepared for her menopause by reading about it. Even though she thought her symptoms were relatively mild, knowing she wasn't going crazy made it easier for her to recognise and deal with them. She said, 'I lived in a hot country [Ghana] and so what some may experience as a hot flush or night sweats was for me just the result of the heat.' At the same time, she had close friends on the other end of the scale. One of her best friends took to changing her nightgown several times a night because she would often wake up drenched in sweat. Other friends became depressed and would no longer join the social events they had always participated in. Noting this, Mum made an even more conscious effort to socialise and stay connected with her peers. She thinks family members should be more aware of how women can experience feelings of isolation and depression during the menopause, and should take extra care to connect with women at this stage of their lives. She pointed out that a number of friends in their fifties became widowed and had to deal with menopause while suddenly bereft of partnership and support, often becoming solely responsible for raising children on their own.

The conversation makes me think of how I need to plan for my own fast-approaching menopause with the same mix of pragmatism and humour that my mum deploys.

For so long my one fear of growing older was that I would no longer be considered sexually attractive or desirable. In the past few years, I have interviewed a number of older women for my book *The Sex Lives of African Women*, as well as for my podcast, *Adventures From the Bedrooms of African Women*, and those conversations have helped me put that fear to bed. Older women have spoken to me about having great sex lives, feeling desired by others, and being full of a sexual confidence that they certainly didn't have in their younger days.

That was not the case for my mum. When I asked her, 'So once the menopause started, did you notice any changes in terms of your sexuality?' she responded: 'Yes, I wasn't interested in sex at all. I had to be convinced and cajoled. And it didn't bother me because I already had my children and I wasn't worried that I might not have any more children. If you're a man and not patient, that's when you will step outside to seek your satisfaction.'

One thing my mum and I have in common is that we were both not bothered about the loss of our fertility. In her case this was because she already had three biological children, and in my case, I only wanted to adopt one child. Where I can see that we're different is how we see sexuality. For me, sex is not about children. It's about pleasure and feeling both desired and desirable, and that's a feeling I want to hold on to for as long as possible. Sex is not something that one does to keep a man from straying: you can't keep men (or any person) from straying if they choose not to stick to the agreements you've made. Sex is something that one does for fun because it feels good and brings feelings of joy and levity.

I don't know how the menopause will affect my sexuality. I know it affects women differently, and that many women feel how my mum did. I also know we live in a world that does not prioritise women's sexual pleasure and so – for many women – sex has always been an obligation: an act that one participates in to please one's partner and/or to have children. I imagine that for those women, the menopause can signify a welcome break: the clearest indication that one is no longer fertile and no longer needs to participate in the performance that sex can sometimes be; a chance to start life free of the encumbrances of men and children, and build oneself anew.

I am excited about being on the road to menopause, hopeful that any physical symptoms I feel will be as mild as those my mum experienced. I am looking forward to throwing away my menstrual cup and embracing days of lounging carelessly on white sheets. I have also benefited from the incredible work that feminists have done on the menopause. I know that there are medical solutions to the very real physical and mental challenges that many women face during the menopause, and I will advocate strongly for myself if I experience these. I know from my mum that I need to keep my band of friends close, and make deliberate efforts to nurture our relationships, and to watch out for those who withdraw. One of the things my mum has deliberately done to keep her mind active has been to read, and I plan to continue reading and writing too: activities that already bring me joy.

Nana Darkoa Sekyiamah (she/her) is the author of *The Sex Lives of African Women*, which *Publishers Weekly* described as 'an astonishing report on the quest for sexual liberation' in their starred review. It was also listed by the *Economist* as the best book of the year. She is also co-founder of *Adventures from the Bedrooms of African Women*, a website, podcast and festival that publishes and creates content that tells stories of African women's experiences around sex, sexualities and pleasure. In 2022, she was cited by the BBC in its list of one hundred inspirational and influential women from around the world. In 2023, *New Africa* magazine listed her as one of one hundred inspirational Africans.

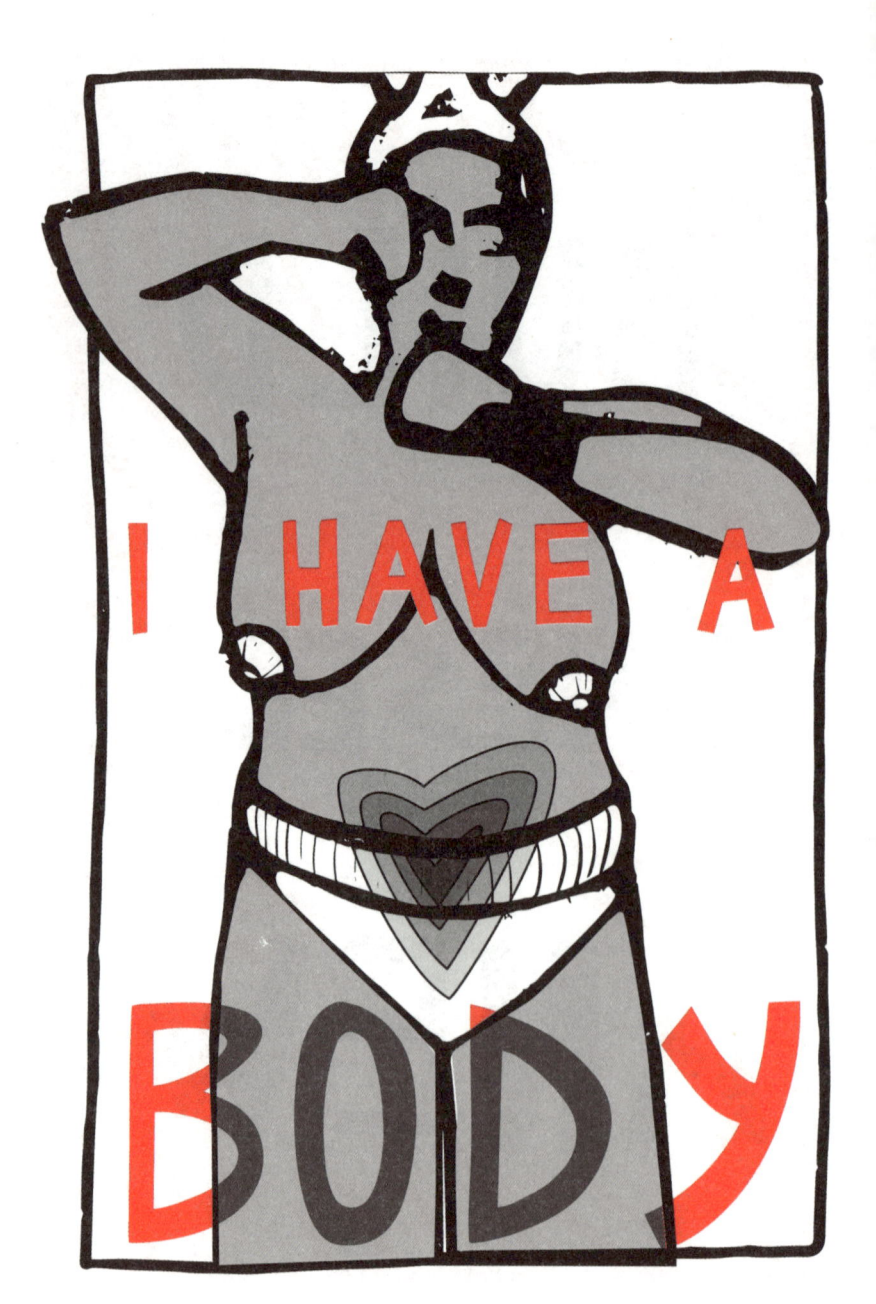

Feeling OldCute. Might Delete Later

Abeer Y. Hoque

1. TICK-TOCK FOR THE COUGARS

I have grown up and grown old with the 'fortune' of looking young-ish. This is partially due to obsessive sunblock use and mostly my non-white ancestors' genes. However, the inexorable process of ageing is now cracking my facade. Take, for example, the time I happened to catch a glimpse of my face in the mirror while doing a forward bend. When you're young, you look the same standing up as upside down. When you're middle-aged, gravity squishes your slackening cheeks against your eye bags, and you look like a clean-shaven Ewok. Or how about no longer being able to rock a cat-eye because your eyelids sag over your handiwork? Sadly, my once lioness hair has thinned to the point that I have to be careful how I claw-clip my hair because that weird cyst/unicorn horn I've been growing for a few years might poke through my mane.

On the physical front of ageing, there are hot flashes, weight gain, vaginal dryness and insomnia. This is on top of the mental Olympics of perimenopause: anxiety, depression, mood swings, brain fog, rage and more. I spent my so-called fertile life bemoaning my period, a recurring scene of blood and pain and moodiness shot through a lens of sexism: fortunes spent on tampons, enduring PMS (premenstrual syndrome) jokes, being barred from entering a mosque. Little did I know that the relief from monthly bleeding would come with so much more, including very dangerous invisible consequences: higher risks of cancer, heart disease and osteoporosis, just to name a few. Damned if I bleed, double damned if I don't.

When I first started experiencing perimenopause, I had no idea what it was. I was forty, had just moved to New York City, and I was feeling anxious. This was a new sensation for me. I have a lot of challenging personality traits. I'm a stubborn, sharp, snap-judgement queen. But I am not an anxious person. My thoughts do not keep me up at night. I am, in fact, a kind of super-sleeper. From my mid-twenties onwards, I eschewed alarm clocks and slept eight hours a night like my life depended on it (it kinda does). I even listed sleep as my religion on the online dating apps.

Don't bother being jealous because I have now joined the 'my thoughts keep me up at night' club, a VIP member, if you will. If something is bothering me, from my partner's inability to put the dish sponge into the sponge house, to my father's descent into the horror that is Alzheimer's, I can't fall asleep or stay asleep or go back to sleep. It's insane-making, and I don't know how you insomniacs have survived this long.

At first, I referred to these episodes as age-onset anxiety, some mysterious dysfunction of getting older. It was only when my period started deviating from its three decades of clockwork rhythm that I realised something else might be going on.

The problem is the general public (including me) barely understands menopause, and we definitely don't tolerate ageing. One person's normal might be another's nightmare, and the only way a person would even know if they were entering perimenopause is if doctors regularly recorded hormone levels from our thirties onwards (they don't, as a rule).

In the spring of 2022, I turned forty-nine and was swinging wildly between three- and seven-week menstrual cycles. I was also having hot flashes half a dozen times a night, leaving me as drenched as if I were standing under a shower. What was astonishing was how quick they were. I'd wake from deep slumber and not know why, and then I would feel it: a rising heat in my chest that would grow until my face was slick, collarbones pooling. Five minutes later, I was at a normal temperature again and would fall back into an uneasy sleep. Until the next heat wave. The only upside (yes, I'm one of those people who keeps a gratitude journal) was I was rarely cold any more.

There were other issues. My body was drying up top to bottom, from my scalp to my eyeballs to my skin to my vagina. For the first three, I resorted to hair oil, eye drops and Vaseline. But the last, my dry vagina, was accompanied by a reduced sex drive, and both were ruining my life. All through my twenties and thirties, I had had a teenage boy's libido. I masturbated once, twice a day, and was that person who wanted sex even during a fight, maybe because of the fight. I had also never used lube. Was I the same person if I didn't desire as much? Was I really turned on if I wasn't wet? Was this what they meant by a midlife crisis? It felt deeply existential but with none of the young hotties in fancy cars.

True to selfish human form, where you only know a good

thing once you've lost it, I have resolved to find a better way to think about ageing. This is a tall order for the deeply ageist society that we live in (double trouble if you're femme presenting). But I couldn't just keep counting my youthful blessings because these were running out fast.

Now, I am not claiming I've figured it out. Ageing is an immemorial intersectional existential mindfuck, and me, I only just figured out how to use a hairdryer in my late forties. The following are merely my thoughts and prayers for ageing gracefully. Or as the writer and director Kaye Cleave calls it, ageing disgracefully, because I'm pretty sure they mean the same thing.

2. THE DREAM OF HRT

By now, many of us in the US have read the February 2023 *New York Times* article[1] on menopause which discusses the benefits of hormone replacement therapy. And we know that this is not a new game. However, a certain flawed, limited and poorly communicated study called the Women's Health Initiative persuaded doctors and their patients to stop hormone replacement therapy (HRT). It's crazy how *The Today Show* can affect the lives of millions in America, but that's exactly what happened in 2002. My mother watched the HRT segment on her TV in Pittsburgh and was terrified by the statistics glibly related on the show. For example: the risk of heart disease and invasive breast cancer increasing by 26–29 per cent. Any statistician can tell you that increasing the risk of breast cancer by 26 per cent is not as bad as it sounds. The risk of breast cancer for those under sixty is 2.33 per cent, and HRT would raise that risk to 2.94 per cent. Or as the *NYT* article puts it, that means eight more cancer patients out of 10,000 people on HRT.

But no one explained any of that to my mom or any of the other non-statistician viewers. She was fifty-four at the time and two years into a very effective course of HRT. She immediately halted the meds, as did tens of thousands, with or without consulting their doctors. And. She. Suffered. For. Years. Joint pain, night sweats, mood swings, the (tangible) works.

Twenty years later, a year before the *NYT* article was published, my younger sister would become the de facto menopause expert in her circle of friends and colleagues in Philadelphia. Ever the overachiever, she had beat me to perimenopause, plus she had read all the original source papers and the follow-up studies, and she had listened to Menopause Barbie's highly regarded podcast (strongly recommend).

By the time the *NYT* article came out, I had already heard the science from my sister, like how people under sixty were significantly under-represented in the original HRT study, which is quite unfortunate, given we were the age group with perimenopause symptoms. She had also explained the benefits of plant-based diets and various herbal supplements, how lifting heavy weights combats the loss of bone density, why it's great to eat dark chocolate, meditate regularly and, my own personal favourite, dance every day. Her painstaking research led her to firing two of her (young, female) doctors before finally finding a third who would even discuss HRT. It should not be this hard.

Two hours north, my own (fifty-plus, female) primary-care physician in Jackson Heights told me that my mother and grandmother before me had likely had perimenopause symptoms, and it was to be expected. Like I was some freshman getting hazed by the oldest (literally) sorority in the world, and I simply had to take it like a woman. Was she even aware of the giant femme-shaped (vaginal?) gap in medical and societal knowledge? I followed my sister's lead and left that practice.

To combat the desert down there, I tried some expensive vaginal lubricating suppositories I learned about on Instagram. But when one little lozenge didn't melt completely, it felt like there was an extra visitor during sexy times, so I stopped. As luck would have it, I found a gynaecologist in Manhattan who calls herself the Vagina Whisperer. She stepped in and prescribed a vaginal oestrogen cream that kinda works. However, this was also around the time my prodigal period returned with a viscous vengeance, so who knows who the real heroine was.

To add insult to injury, despite never having had children, I started experiencing urinary incontinence. Like, not a lot and not that often, and I'd get to the toilet in time, but then my body couldn't wait for my undies to come down and had to serve an aperitivo of pee. I mean, really . . . could we have held out two fucking seconds longer?

My sister is not the only researcher in the family, TYVM. I had a possible solution gleaned from my own studies, although I hadn't been looking up this particular pissing indignity. Some years ago, when I was still a slick sex machine, I had acquired a set of weighted kegel balls. I had gone down the rabbit hole of sex blogs (pun intended) and learned that using these silicon weights might enhance my sexual pleasure. Who doesn't want more of that? Except when I went to research which balls to buy, every review on Amazon was by mothers suffering midlife urinary incontinence, and they were *raving* about the results. Turns out pelvic-floor exercises are good for a lot of things, pornographic and pee-related.

The kegel balls had languished unused for years in my nightstand under my aforementioned gratitude journal and a pile of eye masks and ear plugs. I dug them out, lubed them up as directed and inserted them. It felt weird but I was determined, pairing thirty minutes of weighted kegels with my morning yoga routine, because why not a two-fer? Work out the outside and the inside at once.

3. LESSONS FROM A MONKEY MIND MEDITATOR

Caveat: my meditation practice is about three years young, and I still can't hold focus for more than thirty seconds without thinking about my to-do list. However, I am great at gists and have never been shy about talking, despite very little expertise (thank you, business school and all my white male friends for leading the way). So here are two ideas gleaned from meditation that might help with growing older with ease and joy.

Despite having a fairly healthy body image (given the tragic, front-loaded bell curve of female body images), I had been metering my fatty food intake since I was a teenager. I wasn't counting calories (any more), but I was constantly accounting to the diet goddesses. Two samosas today, none for the rest of the week. Bottomless brunch on Sunday, cereal for dinner. Skip the risotto so I can down three gin and tonics.

Don't ask how many (hundreds of) calories are in a cup of risotto. It's obscene.

I didn't even know how obsessive a food accountant I was until I read Emily Nagoski's excellent book, *Come As You Are* (should be required reading for everyone). In the chapter about increasing your sexual pleasure, Nagoski discusses the tyranny (and uselessness) of diets, in comparison to a more positive lifestyle: Health at Every Size (HAES). What I got out of that chapter was that sexual pleasure was linked to how much you liked your body. It made sense: if you loved your body, you'd have better sex. And sure, I loved my body, but I also wanted it to be a little firmer, thinner, stronger, toneder . . . all the '–ers' and then some. What if (and this was a biggie) I let all of that go? I could still exercise and eat healthy, but maybe I could occasionally eat a cupcake the size of my head and not have to ransom some future pleasure.

It took me a year, dear reader, to finally shut the judgemental food diary in my brain. The year was filled with a million moments of, 'Ah, I'm making a calculation. I'm gonna stop and just try to enjoy this thing I'm putting into my face.' In meditation lingo, this is called 'noting'. I noted and noted and noted again, until finally, at some point I just enjoyed the thing I was eating.

To extrapolate, one way to age (dis)gracefully might be to note when I'm not: when I compare the now to before-times, when I'm harsh with present me, when I despair about future me.

Side note: some of you might be wondering if it 'worked' – did my sexual pleasure increase when I stopped food accounting? Well . . . my partner and I enjoy happy-hour sex. He's a night owl and insomniac, so mornings are his kryptonite. I like to start winding down for bed by 11 p.m., when he might just be starting a movie. So the golden hour is our sweet spot for sexy times. Which sounds all cute, but darlings, there is a *lot* of light, and I used to be tortured with how illuminated my body flaws were. And now I'm more taken with how the sun pours down like honey on me, lady of the hour. So yeah, maybe I am increasing my sexual pleasure.

But then what? What do I replace that ageist taskmistress of time and decrepitude with? Lesson two from meditation is compassion: for that taskmistress and her subject (you). There's a story I heard recently about a Tibetan monk who was captured and held prisoner for twenty-five years. When he finally escaped, a reporter asked him if he had been afraid for his life. And he replied no, but he had been afraid that he might lose compassion for his captors. Yes, I know. That monk is better than all of us combined. But I haven't stopped thinking about it since. Here's my theory: the story is closer to home than we realise. You don't have to channel a Tibetan monk with mountains of fortitude and love. You are already the monk. And you are her captor too.

Our body is our home in the world. It will carry us to the end of our days, fat to wrinkle to fairy dust. Our ideas about age are our prison, but one protecting us from the very real and painful societal trials of being older and femme. Sorta like beating ourselves up before anyone else does. So please, let's forgive ourselves these impossible rules. We don't have to do away with them immediately, or at all, as long as we recognise that they exist because we thought they were helping us.

Being aware that I (body and personhood) am separate from my thoughts (philosophy and society) is the first step.

Loving both parts for what they mean is the second. Feeling free is the final frontier, and I'll get to that in a second. But first, what about beauty, you ask? What about the goddamned loss of it as we get older? That's a hard one, because we're all drinking from the same fountain of forever young. But I'm betting you didn't love everything about being a nubile young thing. So maybe some of those other things got better. For example, my oil-slick skin has finally dried to the point of not having to worry about cystic acne, like I did through my teens and thirties. My twenties were zit-free because I was on birth-control pills, which also made me suicidal. I am only half joking when I say I am hard pressed to choose which was worse. Those of you who've had bad acne know what I mean.

Schadenfreude about our younger selves will only take us so far. So here's a bigger-hearted approach. I've always been better at finding beauty and good in others than myself, so I have been looking hard and kind at older people. It's like the opposite of the time I went on a deplorable Tumblr scroll of thigh gaps, and after about a hundred photos, it started to look horrifyingly normal and I had to stop. Now I scroll the elders, IRL and online. I do it obsessively, regularly, and I note everything I love. It's what the professor and author Savala Nolan calls 'Vitamin Normalise'. For older folks. I promise if you do this, ageing starts to look gorgeously normal. Perhaps not enough to forgive your own face in the mirror, but closer.

4. A MAGIC WAND

So, back to feeling free ... perhaps the most important key to feeling oldcute. Our fear of getting older isn't 'just' about getting wrinkly or injured or ill. It's also about the fear of dying. Remember how forever you felt at twenty-one? And how much more mortal everything feels now? Well, here's one last (literal) magic wand: psychedelics.

These ancient indigenous medicines are starting to be recognised in allopathy for their mental health benefits: from end-of-life panic disorder to grief to depression to anxiety to addiction, and more. Psychedelics are non-addictive, and even the most intense trip will fade in hours. If you're still not convinced, please watch the Michael Pollan documentary *How to Change Your Mind* on Netflix. The second episode is about mushrooms, and it convinced even my Bangladeshi Muslim immigrant mother to try them (that story is for another essay). There's additional research that links chronic physical pain to mental processes, so this dank magical spore could potentially heal your hellish back pain, as it did mine last summer.

Part of what I love about psychedelics is that they are a kind of shortcut to some of the gifts of meditation. You have no choice about being present when you're tripping. You can only be in the here and now when the landscape intensifies its colours, when the ground breathes under you, when you can't stop looking at your own two beautiful hands. I was in the bathroom at a New Year's Eve party last year and saw a magazine cover with a model wearing a poofy pink dress. Under my bewitched gaze, the dress started frothing to epic proportions. It bubbled and spun like cotton candy, frothing right off the page. Did I spend too much time in the bathroom giggling in delight? No, fellow traveller, I wish I had laughed longer.

So the microdoses are helping with my age-onset anxiety, the lessons from meditation are easing the process of ageing, the creams and drops are helping with the desertification of my body. But fuck, the hot flashes are still awful. They sweep in for weeks at a time, disrupting my sleep and sweat-drenching my pjs. I long to be a super-sleeper again, so I think it's time to ask the Vagina Whisperer for HRT. In the meantime, since my body is going to stop circulating vital hormones that keep me stable and sane, the least I can do is change my mind about how I feel.

This is how I found myself in the middle of a chat with Consumer Cellular when the shrooms hit. It was as if the sun had switched on, and the rubber tree's leaves were edged with gold. *Everything felt significant.* The Consumer Cellular agent had found the issue with my bill, but it no longer mattered. What mattered was I was in my body, that I had a body. I closed the chat, hugged myself in wonder and said the kind of thing no sober person would say out loud: I HAVE A BODY. And yes, that body is beset by a storm of retreating hormones, but it still lets me dance and write poetry and eat without guilt. Perhaps the next time I have night sweats at dawn, I'll remember all that.

And you, tender one, looking for whatever it is you're looking for, just for a second, close your eyes. Breathe in deep. Feel the kegel balls doing God's work. Breathe out slow. Open your eyes. We live in a world where sunlight falls from the sky. The ordinary is miraculous.

Abeer Y. Hoque (she/her) is a Nigerian-born Bangladeshi American writer and photographer. She likes reverse sexism, happy-hour sex and spreadsheets. Her books include a coffee-table book (*The Long Way Home*, 2013), a linked collection of stories, poems and photographs (*The Lovers and the Leavers*, 2015), and a memoir (*Olive Witch*, 2017). She has won fellowships from the National Education Association, Queens Council on the Arts, New York Film Academy and the Fulbright Foundation, and holds bachelor of science and master's degrees from the University of Pennsylvania's Wharton School of Business, and a master of fine arts in writing from the University of San Francisco. See more at olivewitch.com

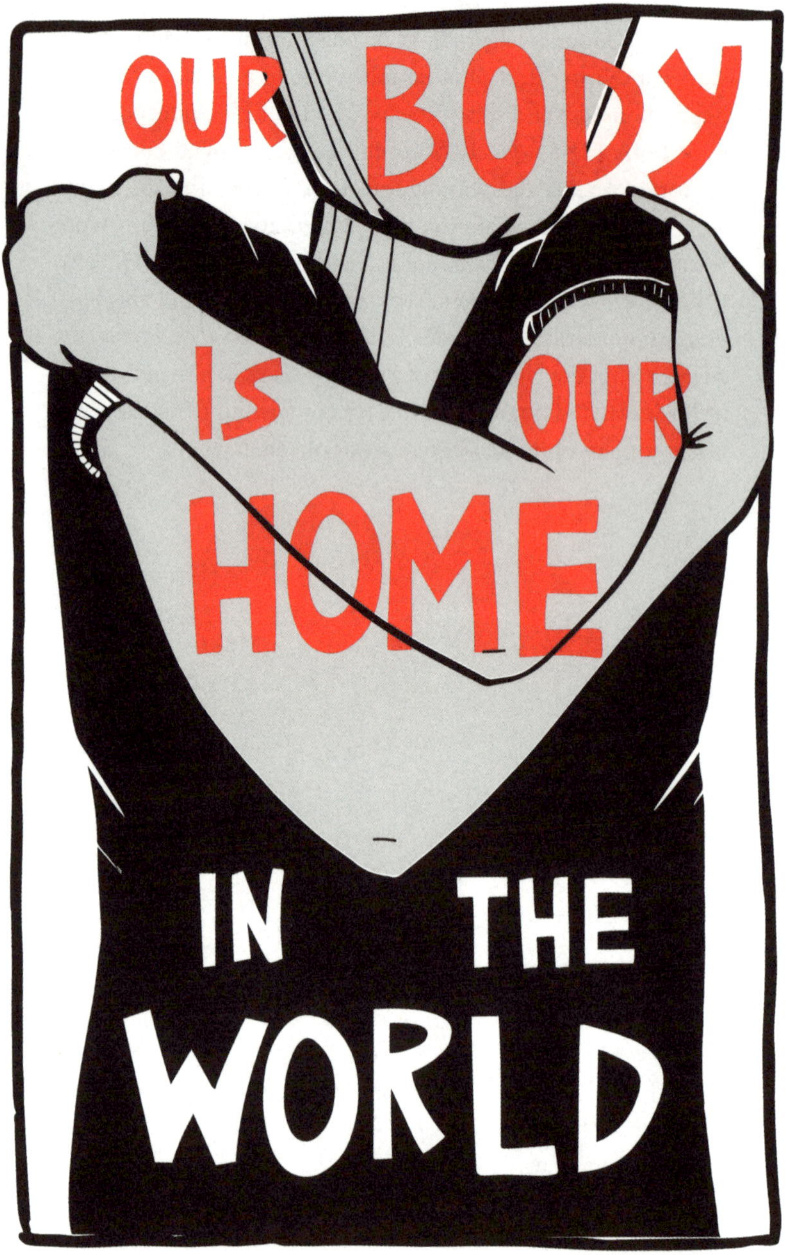
OUR BODY
IS OUR
HOME
IN THE
WORLD

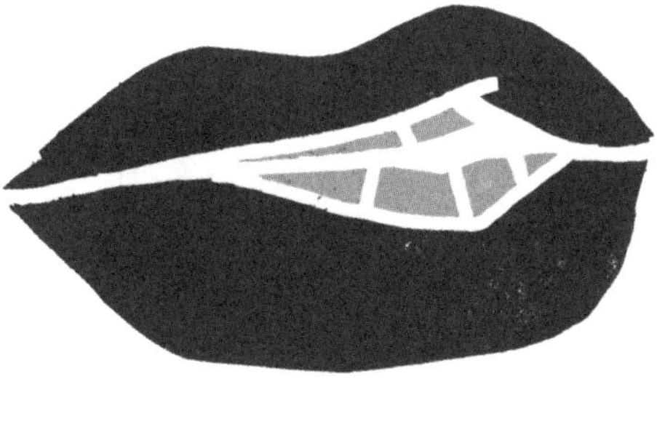

I LONG FOR A ROAD MAP

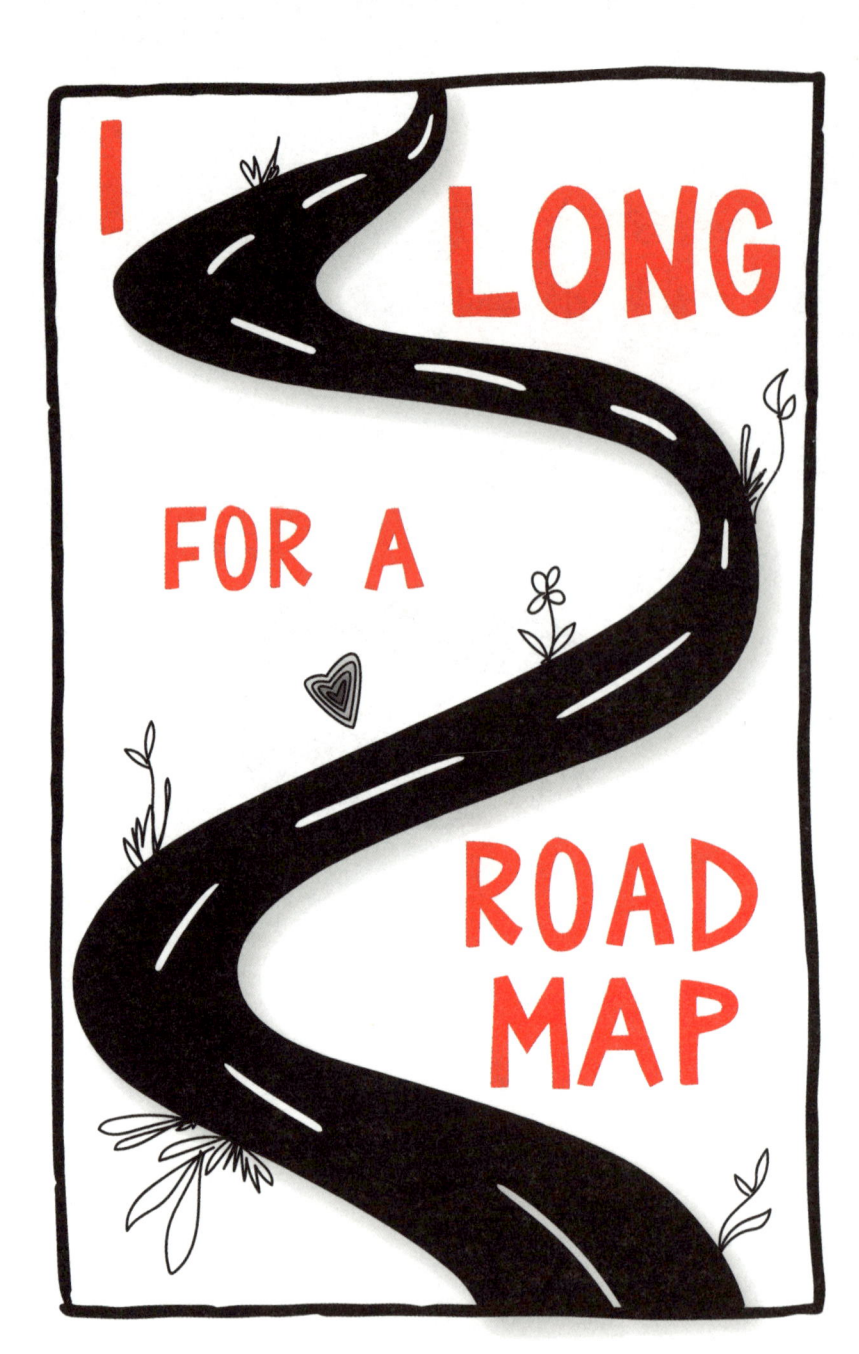

A Field Guide to Menopause

M'kali-Hashiki

As a trauma survivor, I have a back-and-forth relationship with my body. Sometimes I'm extremely present, grounded in this flesh container, aware of every nuance, and sometimes I'm completely unaware of the passage of time. If it wasn't for Facebook, I'd have no way to access my memories of my experiences of menopause. Part of that is definitely the effects of peri/menopause on cognitive skills, but some of that is just me and my PTSD.

I'm fifty-six years old, and thanks to 'Facebook memories' and my iPeriod app, I can say that I've been experiencing perimenopause for about nine years. I feel like I didn't really start paying attention until about five years ago, when my period stopped being regular (it had been highly irregular at first and then had become almost exactly twenty-eight days, starting in my thirties). If menopause is defined by a year of no periods, I'm still stuck in the limbo of perimenopause. It feels like every time I get close to a year, my body decides 'Naw, son' and the hell train starts up again. What did my body give me for my fifty-fifth birthday? A 'gusher': a period with heavy, heavy bleeding. Thanks, body! I have no idea how long I'll be in this 'neither/nor' space, and I'm struggling with how to be fully present within it.

No matter how many twenty- and thirty-somethings refer to me as Auntie, or Teacher, or Miss M'kali-Hashiki (Miss [First Name] is one way that Black folk respectfully address female elders they aren't related to), I just don't think of myself as an elder. And no matter how many seventy-somethings treat me like the young brawn, I know I'm not young either. I feel some days like I'm floundering in place. I want to be present in this time in my life, not thinking wistfully about my 'fertile' years and not rushing ahead to senior citizen.

I have more questions about living in this space than I have answers. Who am I now in this nebulous 'middle age', vs who I was when I was bleeding regularly, vs who I will become once I stop bleeding? What is my place in my community now and then? What's my title? Am I supposed to move into wise elder status suddenly? Can I still get fisted or has my snatch actually shrunk? What is my somatic relationship to the Divine now that my moontime can't be predicted and will eventually end? How do I understand my gender now that the outward markers have changed? I'm just kinda bopping along, questioning, making random posts on my Facebook about what I call perimenopausal roulette and my fucking itchy-ass nipples.

My mama never set me down to prepare me for my period, we didn't have 'the talk'. I started my period at eleven and I do not have fond memories of that time. I grew up with weird shame around my period, like mostly every other middle-class Black girl of my time. It was something to be hidden, to never be discussed. The most embarrassing thing that could happen to you was some sort of evidence that you were currently menstruating. As I came into adulthood, my relationship with my period shifted from 'hidden, shameful, but necessary part of life' to something quite the opposite. While I was never one of those women who felt like my period 'reminded me of the worst part of being a woman', I also wasn't one of those women that painted my lover with my period blood. Yes, I tried free bleeding*, but it just felt 'nasty' to me. I was introduced to the Keeper (the original menstrual cup) at the Michigan Womyn's Music Festival in my early twenties, but I couldn't cut the stem right, so I gave it up. I started using the Instead cups (apparently now called 'menstrual discs'), so over time I got used to seeing and touching and smelling my menstrual blood. And then in my early forties I became a gynaecological teaching associate (GTA) – I taught medical students of all stripes how to do gynaecological exams, using my own body as the demo model. Some weeks I had nine pelvic exams, some weeks I had twenty (most weeks I had none). My first day of work I started my period, and I called my boss to cancel. And she laughed and said, 'I have seventeen women on staff. If I tried to schedule around people's periods, I wouldn't have enough available staff at any given time to fulfil our contracts.' So not only did I become familiar with seeing and smelling my own blood, I became familiar with complete strangers seeing my menstrual blood, my clots; I became familiar with having strangers smelling my blood, seeing me with my menstrual

---

* Free bleeding is when women menstruate without using period products like tampons and pads to catch the period blood.

blood smeared on my thighs, pooling beneath me, or occasionally puddling on the floor. I became adept at discussing menstruation in general and my menstruation specifically without shame. What I'm saying is, I had a very intimate and visceral relationship with my menstrual blood.

And now I don't know when my next period will be, or how long it will last. Sometimes I have PMS symptoms that just go on and on because there's no bleeding to put a stop to them. When my period does happen, I now feel completely incompetent to deal with it. Have tampons changed that much or is it my hoohaw that's so different? Why aren't menstrual discs available globally? Do I remember enough to be able to use this Luna Cup I came across at a store in Cancún? I wouldn't say that I miss bleeding, but I miss that visceral expression of my fertility, of my 'femininity', of my power to produce other living beings. Of the power of my humanity, because there's something awesome and primal about bodily fluids, and I miss being up close with mine on a regular basis. I miss that connection to the moon (I did eventually become synced to the full moon, which delighted my Blitch* heart). As someone who leads erotic moon rituals on the new and full moons, I feel somewhat like one of my magic tools is missing. What will fill the void of that relationship with the moon, or how do I craft a new one?

I entered this liminal space of perimenopause woefully underprepared. Just like Mama didn't prepare me for starting

---

* A slang term that is a portmanteau of 'Black' and 'witch'. It can mean specifically a Black woman/femme who strictly follows Wicca, or it can be a Black woman/femme who incorporates aspects of Wicca or witchcraft into their personal practice. For me, it's the latter.

menstruation, she didn't prepare me for menopause either. All I learned was whatever I could pick up from her conversations with her older sisters or her friends. The main thing that really sticks in my mind is that I remember my oldest aunt called once, and in the course of the conversation, I was able to glean that she was complaining about her period. She was sixty-something, which means that Mama would have been in her fifties, which meant I was in my twenties, and I remember thinking, *Whoa! Forty more years of this?!*

The only thing I knew to expect was hot flashes, gleaned from overheard conversations and pop culture's fascination with mocking women's lived experiences. Truth be told, I was kinda looking forward to hot flashes, because I am/was always cold. That longing went on until I had my first (of thankfully only two hot flashes), and I was blown away by the intensity, and felt so frantic during both of them, knowing to my core that this was completely unsustainable, and I had no idea how some women lived with them for years. My most noticeable and longest-lasting peri/menopause symptom is itchy nipples. For years they were itchy constantly, the kind of itching that makes you think you might be rending your flesh with the ferocity of your scratching, and it's still not enough. Now they're only itchy every now and then, and the sensation doesn't last long enough for me to fear making myself bleed while searching for relief.

My vagina has changed in ways that threaten to unravel my sex life completely. My 'kink' is being penetrated before my body is fully ready, before my vaginal walls have relaxed and ballooned, before my body produces adequate lubrication. That is simply no longer possible without injury. I have been having sex with postmenopausal people for some time now, so I know that the whole 'you're gonna dry up' is not true, but I'm just not producing enough lubrication to have the kind of sex in the ways I used to, and even more store-bought lube is not enough, because the vaginal tissue has actually thinned. Part of my retirement from my gig as a GTA was because I just couldn't handle multiple insertions of a metal speculum in a day. I tried changing the lubricant, which made it more comfortable, but my body decided quite forcefully that we were no longer gonna be doing that job. I loved that job, and I think that I might feel some hidden resentment to my body, to perimenopause for making it no longer doable.

And now it feels like every day some new wacky symptom shows up, and it's just another symptom of peri/menopause. And I just wish there was a manual somewhere that you received at, like, thirty: 'Here's What to Expect When You're Expecting . . . Menopause'. Yes, it's individualised, but there's still enough commonality that we shouldn't be being caught unawares. I don't want to encourage a pathologising of peri/menopause, but I think it would make the whole experience a bit more chill if you had some idea of what you were in for, other than fucking 'hot flashes'.

Prior to the pandemic, I was kinda digging my perimenopausal state. I was having the best sex of my life. I was more in my body than in my younger days (only some of it due to therapy). About seven years ago I started being able to orgasm from penetration alone, which is great, not because I think that heteronormative expectations have any place in my sex life, but because it means it takes less effort for me, I have to use fewer muscles, and I don't have to worry about orgasm headache.

And now I'm not digging it as much. My body is becoming so unfamiliar, after me spending so much time working through my PTSD to fully inhabit it. I'm tired of freaking out about some symptom, only for a doctor to tell me it's a common thing for 'women my age'. If it's so goddamn common, why the fuck didn't I know about it? Why is this time of life glossed over? Why does popular culture depict femininity as 'nubile prepubescent' to 'hot twenties' to 'motherhood' and then a sort of blank spot, straight to 'grandmahood'? Perimenopause is that blank spot and I wish there was a little, no, a lot more light shone on it.

I haven't had sex with another person since before the pandemic, so when I think about my libido, it's in reference to self-pleasure only. My libido is pretty low these days, but I'm almost positive it has nothing to do with perimenopause. I'm almost positive it's low cuz we're still in a fucking pandemic and so many people are showing just how fucking selfish they are, how much they think me and mine are disposable offerings on the altar to capitalism, so being in a general state of arousal just from being alive hasn't been a place I've occupied in a while.

My understanding of my gender is not 'changing' exactly: I'm still a woman and I still feel like a woman, but I have to rely so much on that bedrock of inner knowing in a different way than before, because the outward markers of my 'femininity' have changed. We are in a time where we have the opportunity to have a deeper understanding of our gender as cis women, divorced from our plumbing. And that opportunity is even more evident to me as my hormones shift and my body changes and I face the more than likely removal of my uterus (80 per cent of Black women will experience fibroids in their fifties, and are up to three times more likely than white women to have surgery because of it[1]). I feel like, for cis women, mainstream depictions of menopause include a sort of neutering or de-womanising. Because society has so conflated womanhood with 'fertility' and things like 'bodily hairlessness', and all sorts of external markers that change so much during this time. I'm also realising how much of 'womanhood' is tied to external factors like 'how fuckable I'm perceived to be'. Mostly how fuckable men perceive me to be, but even in the queer world, femmeness (related to but not the same as 'femininity') is in some cases defined by how attractive you are to other queers. And attractiveness is still tied to youth, or the outward markers of it, which can be manufactured.

One of my friends mentioned that we are the first generation to still have a good twenty to thirty years postmenopause. I don't know if I think that's true (my maternal aunts are both long-lived and entered menopause pretty late). What I think is true is that we are the first generation to be postmenopausal and still focused on self. I do not have children or grandchildren, and I have no blood siblings (my niblings are all children of the siblings of my heart). My life right now is very much focused on my own contentment and fulfilment: my work, my writings, my spiritual development, my travel. I can do that because I don't have the same type of obligations that my mama, my aunts or Big Mama (my grandmother) had at this age. What does it mean to claim this stage of life without being focused on 'nurturing' or 'guiding' younger people? Self as priority is always directly or indirectly punished if it's a woman living it.

What is my title? I'm not a crone (that just feels way too white of a label), I cringe when someone refers to me as 'ma'am' and I shuddered the first time a child called me 'Miss M'kali-Hashiki'. I'm trying on 'Auntie' for size. It still doesn't feel right, but I'm trying. I remember joking after the *Verzuz** with Patti LaBelle and Gladys Knight that maybe the Auntie Rite of Passage involved another auntie just appearing before you with a perfectly tailored pantsuit for you to put on, and then welcoming you to The Circle of Aunties, where y'all just go eat turkey necks, collards, pound cake and endless vats of mac and cheese while drinking Henny and Coke without spilling anything on your impeccable pantsuit.

I hate the way I look in pantsuits.

I recently bought a pair of Doc knock-offs and some new dresses, and when I showed a friend a pic of my outfit, she said I looked like an anime warrior, which I think is the best compliment anyone has paid me in a long time. In my mental image I still wear the punk/New Wave outfits of my youth. I miss having hair colour not found in nature, but I also like my grey. I am convinced that an undercut is a global sign of queerness and as I travel through Latin America, I want to express my queerness, but more subtly. So I compromised with blue hair that doesn't cover all my gray, and I have a side shave instead of an undercut.

I don't know what 'dressing my age' even means any more, but I'm not ready for pantsuits.

We really are in a different time than those who most recently came before us who we might have looked to in order to understand this particular period (pun intended?) of our lives. We have a broader understanding of gender, we are

---

* A popular webcast series in the US where two stars in the entertainment industry compete with their best hit record.

better able to articulate all the ways in which white supremacist ideals have infiltrated our minds, our bodies, even as consciously we reject them and seek deeper connection with our ancestral lineages.

I long for a roadmap through this liminal space, a roadmap informed by my culture and broadened by my queerness and my 'Gen Xness', but there is not one already prepared. Even as more people speak about peri/menopause, there is no space for my wholeness in those conversations because they're either too white or too straight or too cis (even though I am cis, I don't want cisness to define this roadmap, making it too narrow for me to walk it with all of my community). It is both exciting and daunting to know that we are creating our own map by saying the things white supremacy told us never to say, by sharing the things we are supposed to be too ashamed to show another living being, and by witnessing the things we are supposed to ignore. That we are creating something not only for ourselves, but for those who come after.

With that in mind, I co-created a salon series for QTIBIPOC (Queer, Trans and Intersex, Black, Indigenous, People of Colour) with Taiwanese American healer and writer Syd Yang to talk and listen to our own stories about finding our way through perimenopause. The salons were heavily attended by folx of different ages, genders, ethnicities. And what struck us most intensely was the hunger for community, the hunger for these stories, the affirmation that we are not alone, that what is happening to our bodies and our feelings about those happenings were not unique. There has always been something healing, something powerful about sharing our stories, about learning that our experiences are mirrored by another.

M'kali-Hashiki (she/her) is a somatic storyteller and erotic ritualist. Her divine purpose is helping folx access Eros as a renewable resource in their liberatory and revolutionary toolkits. She offers community journeys, rituals, individual coaching, instructional videos and guided visualisations to help us survive and thrive during these chaotic times. She also offers sexuality training and employee wellness/team-building skills to organisations and companies, and is a skilled sensitivity reader of manuscripts, ensuring avoidance of explicit and implicit systemic bias. Her lived experiences as a fat, Black, queer, femme trauma survivor inform every aspect of her work. More info at FiercePassions.com

IF IT'S SO GODDAMN COMMON, **WHY THE FUCK** DIDN'T I KNOW ABOUT IT ??

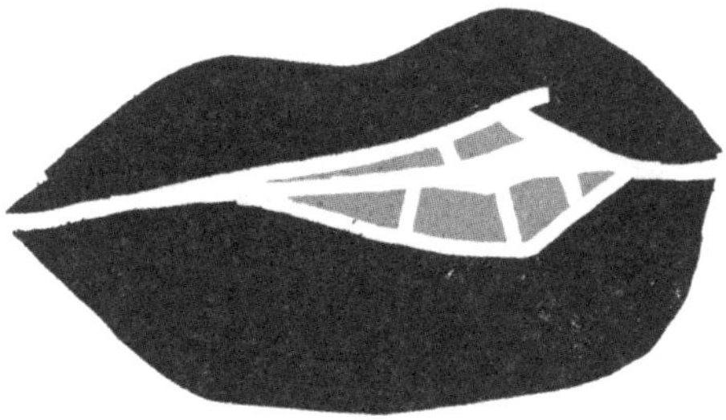

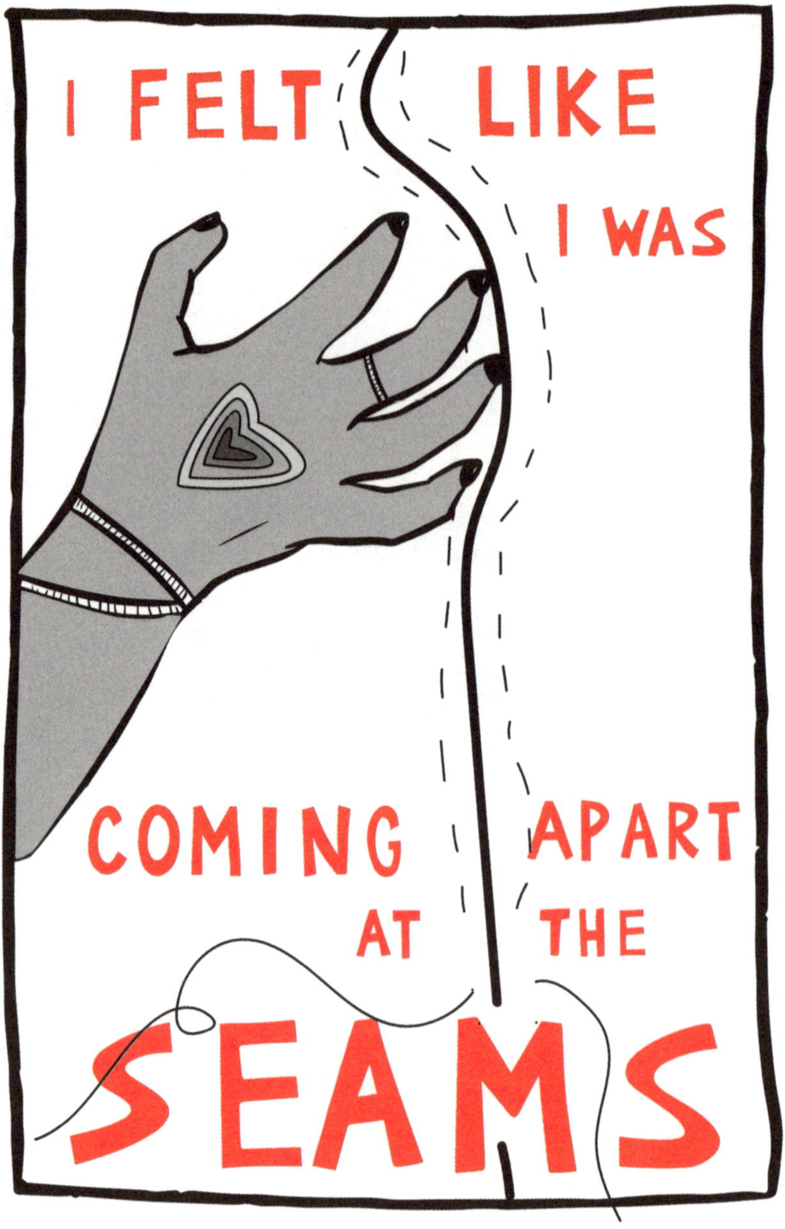
I FELT LIKE
I WAS
COMING APART
AT THE
SEAMS

Free Fall

Syd Yang

'Wake up!' my body screamed at me, urgent waves of a familiar sense of dread coursing through my legs.

'You're about to leak! Don't bleed on the bed!' another voice yelled, yanking the covers off and catapulting me out of the bedroom.

'Fuck.' A single word crashed out of my mouth the moment a river of blood gushed down my legs and pooled onto the tiled floor beneath my feet. My mind was spinning. 'How is this possible?' I had in a menstrual cup and was wearing underwear. How much blood did that have to be to breach these barriers? How angry was my blood in its refusal to be contained any longer?

Slowly, I made my way down the hall to the bathroom, still leaking, a trail of blood spattering along the floor. I needed to clean up before I would be able to assess the damage. It was 3 a.m. My cat followed me gingerly down the hall, deftly stepping around the polka dots of red. He stared curiously at me as he sat down next to the shower and watched. Perhaps he was judging – after all, he is a cat. I could only imagine what he was thinking. Blood was everywhere. What horrible crime had just been committed? Blood was smeared on everything. I peeled off my underwear, pulled off my night shirt and began to cry. What was happening to me?

My body would recreate this crime scene three more times over the next several months, twice even in one single night. By the third time I wondered if perhaps 3 a.m. showers were an unexpected pleasure in all of this. There was a sweet joy in letting my body be caressed by hot water in the quiet pause of an early, early morning. The water was helping me surrender to what was.

Up until then my body's bloodletting had been slowing down. For several years my periods had been shortening in duration and the flow was getting lighter (though they never had been that heavy to begin with). About six months before this first sudden flow, I had begun to skip periods altogether. The day before this first crime-scene incident, I had started to bleed again after three months of nothing. I had no idea what was waiting for me.

How had thirty-seven years of bleeding every month not prepared me for this? All of this was unsettling in ways for which I was not prepared. Nothing anyone else had shared with me about menopause had prepared me for this. I did not know how to respond. In the days and months that followed, I scrambled, grasping at whatever information I could find, hoping it would be the magic ripcord that, once pulled, would open a parachute I needed to guide me gently back to solid ground. I needed things to make sense. I wanted it to make sense. Once again in my life, markers of femininity that my body carried sparked chaos and refused to make sense to me.

The reality was sinking in slowly that perhaps there was no parachute – or, rather, I had been dealt a defective one. Just my luck. I was free-falling fast and I also didn't know how to fly.

The first time I fucked a woman while she bled, a vermilion glove coated my hand, guiding me deeper – two fingers, then three, the palm of my hand being pulled down and into sacred space as it curled up into itself.

Blood does not lubricate. It clings and coats and drips down arms, creating layers of connection as bodies rise and fall into each other.

Blood is life force, the nectar of the vampire, the vital elixir that courses through our veins. It is identity, it is culture, it is purpose and it is a reminder of who we are.

A parachute is a lifeline between the sky and the earth, an intermediary between the unpredictability of the wind and the stability of terra firma. One puts on a parachute before leaping out of a plane. A parachute presumes forethought, the intentionality of planning for a known event. A parachute has one job – to hold someone as they fall. Who or what was holding me as I fell? I knew this was coming – why was there no parachute ready for me?

As a young adult, I lost community. I lost family. I lost access to elders. I lost care from older women who could have offered me wisdom and support when menopause would show up in my life. Coming out as queer (and later, nonbinary/transmasculine) within the world I was raised in – one that shaped itself around evangelical Christianity – created irreparable fractures and severed most of my relationships at that time. I had to figure out how to survive alone in a body that didn't always make sense, that wasn't supposed to thrive in the world (as I was led to believe). How was I supposed to find care for a body that continues to be systematically pathologised in both the political and medical spheres?

Being in a free fall without a parachute wasn't new. Without reference points and trusted elders to show me how to construct a viable parachute, I convinced myself then that free-falling might be a form of flying. I would be OK. I had to be OK. Even so, my blood continued gushing out. I had already been pushed out of the plane. I had to believe that I was going to be OK, parachute or not.

> *I feed the earth with my blood – spilling out underneath a full moon, mingling with the soil that grows the medicines we crave in order to survive.*
>
> *I have placed my blood in cauldrons, smeared it on parchment, hands stained crimson as I call up the power of the Great Mother to heal me, to hold me, to save me.*
>
> *I got my first period when I was eleven, a sledgehammer to the gut as my mother dragged me out in front of the women in church to brag about how I now bled.*
>
> *'Isn't this so exciting?' she exclaimed, my eyes locked in a wide horror as a mass of disembodied hands reached out to pat me on the head, to claim access to a body that had betrayed me – a body that would take me many more years to embrace.*

'My body is betraying me!' I told my acupuncturist a few years before I would learn to love 3 a.m. showers. I unleashed a deluge of bodily complaints. 'My body feels untethered!

Like I'm being tossed about in a hurricane and I've lost track of how I'm supposed to feel. Nothing makes sense.'

I was in my early forties and this acupuncturist was the only elder Chinese woman I had a trusted relationship with at the time. She laughed, lovingly shook her head at me as she proceeded to silently puncture the skin of my body with thin needles, over and over again.

'Rest. You'll be fine. But also know that it will get much worse when you turn fifty.' Without breaking into a smile this time, she stared at me for a beat then walked out. I was left alone with my body, asking dozens of needles to teach me how to fly. I didn't even know then I could have been asking for a parachute.

But these days.

These days, I am bleeding less and less, an ageing uterus fluffing blankets and ironing sheets, preparing itself for a coming rest.

Blood is the giver of life, a well-aged wine trapped within the Holy Grail, a secret held by elusive knights sworn to keep her safe.

My blood is boiling, large gasps of air rising through my arteries as I read the news these days.

'America First?' my blood screams, as all my white blood cells rise up to destroy the echo of a white-supremacist chant. My red blood cells hold the circle, standing guard, the lions at the doorway, teeth bared, nostrils flared.

My forty-seventh birthday had just passed. My body was, once again, becoming an unfamiliar guest in my life. What was happening? I couldn't sleep. I could barely remember words I had just said, let alone a thought that passed through my mind. My irritability refused to be contained. The recurrent headaches I had suffered from a few years back were showing up again, this time with an unrelenting vengeance. Almost daily, I was forced to lie down, cancel meetings and turn out the lights. Something was off. I was untethered, free-falling again. This time around, a new edge emerged as my anger grabbed the reins and was running the show.

I was going through a divorce at this time. My periods were getting lighter still but remained annoyingly regular. Maybe it wasn't perimenopause at all, it was just grief wreaking havoc on my body? I felt like I was coming apart at the seams. Grief was taking me out, and even so, perimenopause must have still been operating lightly in the background, right? All I know for certain is that I was getting older. But no, it must have been the grief. That's what I was telling myself. The body discomfort and dissonance couldn't be anything else. Get past my grief and I would feel better. That had to be the answer.

Grief and perimenopause are not good playmates. My anger was turning in on myself and it didn't feel easeful at all. I must have done something wrong for it to be this bad. Maybe I was falling apart because I couldn't figure out how to be good enough to be loved. Was that it? I struggled with discerning between fact and fiction so much of the time. All the brain fog, the emotional chaos and body discomfort must have been because I was doing something wrong – because I didn't have a parachute (everyone else had one, though, right?).

I checked in with my primary-care physician for an annual well-body exam. I longed for answers, desperate now for a parachute to save me. She conducted a pap smear, asked all the way too personal, irrelevant questions and then I prompted her about perimenopause. 'Could this be what's going on?'

'Oh, you're fine,' she dismissed in a flippant tone, 'but, you know, if you lose some weight, you'll probably feel better.'

> *This is my blood memory rising, the flow of generations of those who resisted, the flow of women who were unwilling to be silenced, the flow of communities whose power refused to be erased.*
>
> *Mixed-race, I carry a dissonant chorus of memories within me. Today, it is the blood of the witches and druids who stood up to the Catholic oppressors of Rome, the blood of the Indigenous Taiwanese whose names were stolen from the family tree, and the blood of a lineage of women silenced by addiction and abuse, that respond to the fire within.*
>
> *These are the memories boiling up within me, steam compressed within my heart releases the dragon's fire.*
>
> *My blood memory calls me forward, reminds who I am, begging me to never forget.*

The intersection of grief and perimenopause opened up a portal in my body that I was being invited to walk through. Did I have a choice, I wondered? Perhaps I would find my parachute on the other side? Maybe this could be the doorway that would teach me how to fly?

People say that when you are about to die, your entire life flashes before your eyes. I'd like to revise that. A life deconstructing while my body was free-falling through discomfort and confounding change was the screen upon which I could watch my entire life replay before me. What needed to die for me to get to the other side of menopause? Questions plagued me. Existential angst had become the friend who never left me alone. Who am I? Why am I here? Where am I going? What do I even know any more?

> *I am bleeding less and less these days, the life-creator within me getting ready for her final bow, her closing performance already winking at me from the nearby horizon.*
>
> *I have eaten the blood of chickens and pigs, congealed into squares of metallic sweetness, floating in a bowl of soup.*
>
> *I have drenched the white sponge of a hand-torn chunk of bread in the pink ribbons dripping off of a steak knife, and I have sucked it dry.*

When I first started skipping periods, I began to notice an unfamiliar freedom in my body that felt so welcome. I was less angry. Ease was unexpectedly creeping in – and it wasn't from anything I was consciously doing to make things better. Was I allowed to be happy about this? Was this supposed to feel this good? Menopause was about losing out on life, right? Didn't this mean I was becoming less attractive, less able to find love again, less viable as a human being in the world? These are some of the stories that had crept into my body over the years, distracting me from a sense of self-worth. Even so, menopause was offering me a freedom I never believed was possible in a body that housed a uterus.

Not-bleeding was powerfully gender-affirming, I discovered. In the ever-lengthening gaps between blood flows, my breath found more time to rest. My body was becoming more spacious. I was beginning to exhale in ways that allowed my shoulders to widen and my feet to root deeper into the ground beneath me. New choices in this body were becoming possible.

Gender had been both a known and a not-yet-fully-known entity my entire life. As a child I fought to change my name to be gender-neutral (I lost that fight with my parents) and I gave up wearing dresses by the time I was ten. Internally I struggled for years with what it meant to be a woman – was I doing it right? What was I missing? Why was so much of what I was told was special about femininity so confounding and uncomfortable for me? My body must be wrong. I must be wrong. I must be doing something wrong.

I first got my period when I was eleven. I was devastated. I hated that this was happening, but I couldn't necessarily articulate why. Each time I bled in the many years that followed, I got angry. Rageful, even. My blood was angry, always so angry.

'That's just PMS,' everyone told me. 'Stop being so emotional.'

I knew it was something more, but I didn't yet fully know what that might be.

My period felt like an alien visitation each time that it showed up. 'I'm not from this world, your world, but here I am. Deal with it.' My period never felt necessary; it was a nuisance. 'Go away!' I retorted.

What was the point, even? Every month I engaged in this internal battle. Over the years I resigned to this irritation as something I would just have to endure. I kept telling myself,

'This is the body you were born into. You have a uterus. Deal with it.'

In my mid-twenties I asked myself if perhaps I wanted to take testosterone, as many of my transmasculine friends were doing. 'It will stop the bleeding,' they promised. I was intrigued, and yet each time I checked in with my body, it said, 'Nope. Testosterone is not our path right now.' This felt like body wisdom, so I listened.

If I was going to be resigned to deal with monthly blood, then I was determined to stay angry, which I did.

> *I am bleeding less and less these days, the whistle of the elder getting louder in my ear each month.*
>
> *'Come to me,' they sing, a wisp of grey hair floating past my eyes.*
>
> *'I'm not ready,' I whisper back, blood still clinging to the grooves of my fingernails, even after I have washed my hands.*

Perhaps it was the perimenopause, perhaps it was healing from profound grief and the wounds born out of decades of emotional abuse in my relationships. Perhaps it was something else altogether. Wisdom was rising in my body as I wandered through my forties, and I began to hear a new, seductive whisper beckoning me down a new path. 'It's time.' My body spoke gently to me, first in the form of dreams and later as it wove into an embodied knowing in my waking consciousness. 'It's time.'

By my forty-ninth birthday I had added an endocrinologist to my healthcare team. That morning, I held testosterone in my hands, my body anxious to begin walking this new path. With each day that passed, my testosterone levels rose, eventually reaching a plateau where it hangs out now, mirroring typical 'male' levels. The anger that my blood carried so loyally has almost fully dissipated and my body continues to shape-shift into a more honest version of itself. These days, I continue to discard masks and costumes I no longer feel obligated to wear. I am becoming more whole in the most spiritual of ways possible. I no longer remember the last time I bled. My uterus is resting, finding more appropriate ways to bide its time.

What if my uterus was never meant to bleed? What if my menopause is less about what is 'ending' and more about what is 'beginning'? What if my uterus's biological imperative was to remind me how to give birth to divinity rather than another human being? What if perimenopause was not a crisis at all, rather a rebirthing process into more manifest forms of my inherent nobility?

I am bleeding less and less these days, the ancestors in my blood calling their memories back to them. Soon, I will bleed no more, my flow turning inwards, my life-force no longer for others to consume.

I will be nurturing new blood memories for the next generations, for those yet to come.

My blood is getting ready to become the blood of a wise being, the one who will first prick the finger of the Devil instead of their own.[1]

Perimenopause, for me, was about contradictions. It was about travelling the unknown roads, choosing the unfamiliar paths. It unravelled everything I thought I knew – about myself, about life, about relationships, about possibility. It reinforced for me that I am not a woman, that gender is more expansive and mysterious than I may ever be able to explain. It has taught me that I can absolutely trust the body I reside within, that wisdom is carried inside me that stretches back generations and will reach forward into all that will be. My body is not wrong. It never has been and it never will be.

The parachute I had been searching for has always been here with me. It is my body itself – in its profound sacredness and in its delicious wholeness. I never needed to know how to fly. I simply needed to be called home into a body that walks this magnificently mind-boggling and exhilarating life alongside me.

Syd Yang (they/them) is a mixed-race (Taiwanese and European American) queer/trans writer, Buddhist chaplain/minister and spiritual-care practitioner who weaves together magic, prayer and intention in the world through their practice, Blue Jaguar Healing Arts. Their work locates its resonance at the intersections of memory, body, sexuality and mental health. More at bluejaguarhealingarts.com

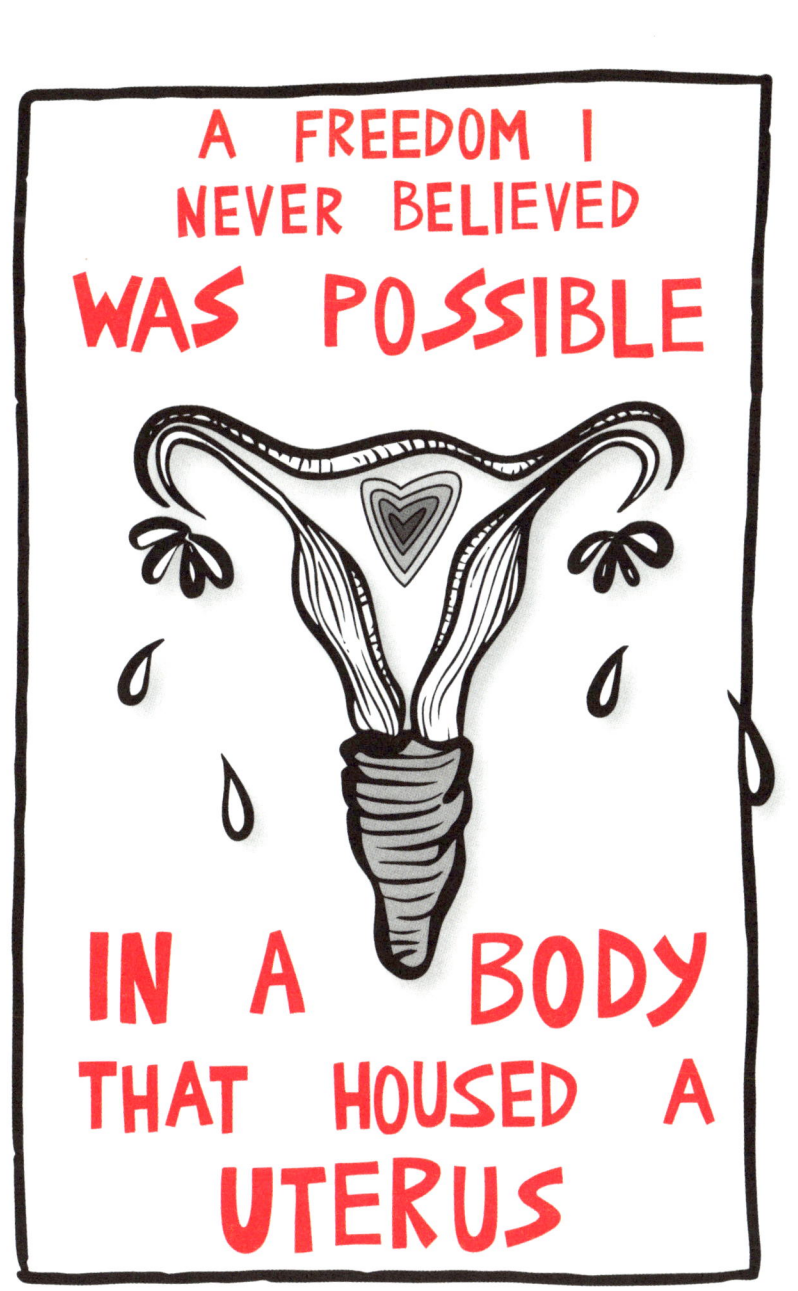

A FREEDOM I NEVER BELIEVED WAS POSSIBLE IN A BODY THAT HOUSED A UTERUS

Afterword

Menopause fucked me sideways.

First it went for my vagina.[1] Then it came for my words. Sex and writing. Oof. It felt particularly cruel for menopause to be so fucking bespoke: to so fashion its challenges to fit exactly what I feared the most.

(I'm punching the air right now because I can't remember the last time I enjoyed writing; enjoyed a turn of phrase I came up with that reminded me why I am a writer; that reminded me that I love life.)

This is the first essay I've written in eight months.

I am able to write it because I started menopause hormone therapy (MHT) – something I had long resisted – at the end of January. It has calmed the anxiety that has had me in a chokehold for more than five years, helped me sleep without my nightly dose of CBD (cannabidiol) and/or THC (delta-9-tetrahydrocannabinol). I love cannabis – but I'd rather use it recreationally than necessarily. And in so doing, it has turned my mind from a place deserted of ideas and which no longer welcomed me into a place excited to once again create sentences and weave together thoughts that so excite me that I would pull my phone out on walks to capture my ideas as voice notes. I am lucky because my gynaecologist neither pushed MHT nor withheld it from me. She explained to me my options, patiently and with great detail, just before I became postmenopausal in 2022. I chose at the time not to start MHT. When I told her earlier this year that I could not work or focus and that I felt deflated and wanted relief, she explained the various therapies available to me.

She herself is on MHT, understood immediately when I told her I could not write, and shared her own menopause struggles.

This essay is not to persuade you to start or not start MHT. That is a conversation that I hope you can have with your healthcare provider, and it is a decision that is only yours to make. I want, instead, to continue an openness around my menopause transition,[2] to fracture any shame or stigma around a stage of life for anyone who has ever had a uterus and ovaries. So much of that shame and stigma around the menopause transition is impossible to detangle from sexism and ageism, in a world that is unforgiving to anyone who is not a white, able-bodied and affluent cisgender heterosexual man. To even tiptoe onto the shore of vulnerability in such a world when you are not those things is to invite derision, if you're lucky, and destruction the rest of the time.

There is a reason that so many women leave the workforce during the menopause transition.[3] That reason is why so many who are going through the menopause transition in positions of power say nothing about it.[4] We know how lack of workplace accommodation during the menopause transition can impact career.[5] That is the reason that I am telling you that I have not been able to work and have barely made a living since last summer because of my menopause transition.

I invite derision, destruction and shamelessness that leaves me accountable to no one but a self (mine, me) that I owe a powerful and tender love.

A cisgender woman must be able to say, 'This is hard. This has tested me to the limits,' without being considered weak or worthless in this world built by and for (white, able-bodied and affluent cisgender heterosexual) men.

Since last summer, I have not been able to write anything that is longer than an email or a tweet/Instagram caption or to read anything for pleasure that is longer than a tweet/Instagram caption. I would read essays I'd written in 2020, when I launched FEMINIST GIANT, with wonder and awe. I wrote an essay a week back then! I envied whoever that Mona was and her ability to write so effortlessly. I envied people reading on the subway, wistful for the days I'd miss my station because I was so lost in a book. In 2019, I set and met the challenge of reading a book per week. What? Who was that?!

I became convinced I had read and written so much in those last few years of perimenopause because something within me knew we would run out of words – like Joseph convincing the ancient Egyptians to stock up before the famine. Or an animal preparing to hibernate, stocking up on words like food, as if I knew I would go into a fast from words and I needed to eat all the words to keep me full until the new ones came.

But when? I was terrified. Would they ever return?

It became a challenge to myself to tell anyone who would listen that I was the writer who could no longer write. I was trying to deflate the terror but all I deflated was me. If I did not work for myself, I would have resigned. I effectively did.

I am the writer who foolishly (ambitiously, deliriously) signed on to deliver two books about menopause until she could not – because of menopause.

The first book was this anthology.

Other people wrote it. Easy, right? But I could not read, let alone edit, the essays that an incredible line-up of contributors had delivered to me months earlier. One extension after another allowed me to divide the reading into small chunks until I was finally able to send the book to the publisher. Thank you, Aliya Sultan, for your patience and understanding, and massive gratitude to all the contributors.

It got worse.

A year after signing on to write my third book, *The King Herself: How Hatshepsut Helped Me Unbecome*, I had to confess to my editor that I had not written a single word and that I did not know when I would be able to deliver that memoir of menopause. I had already asked for an extension to the deadline. And I had failed to meet it.

When she called me soon after to offer support and to tell me she was extending my deadline until 2026, I was on the verge of tears in an aisle at Target. A thousand thanks, Rakia Clark. You are my forever editor. You have shown what is the workplace accommodation that so many menopausal people are urging.

And that was the moment I decided to start MHT.

Why did it take me so long?

Initially, my hesitation was because I hated hormonal birth control when I was younger.

A part of me wanted to just keep ploughing through menopause. To just get on with it and be as 'strong' as I know I am.

Until I couldn't.

I wanted to age without interference, for a lack of a better term. And the menopause transition is the memo we all get that we are ageing. Again, I wanted to just slog through it.

Until I couldn't.

A part of me wanted to make it through the menopause transition, with all the fuckery it threw at me, without 'help'. What qualifies as help is where things get interesting: I had used several non-hormonal supplements to address the fuckery that menopause threw at me. How come those weren't 'help'? What was it about hormones that made me feel like I was 'giving up' or 'taking an easy way out'?

I was aware, of course, of the now reassessed study that had led so many women to stop taking hormone therapy during their menopause transition.[6] I also did not want to start taking hormones only to have all the fuckery return again once I stopped taking them. So I thought – tough it out now and it will be better on the 'other side'. But would it? And for how much longer would I be 'toughing it out'?

Please note the quotation marks – I'm quoting my inner Greek chorus/inner critic/any other harsh voice that makes you feel like shit. Let me show you how it works.

I expected the wonderful acupuncturist I was seeing to judge me when I told her that I was considering going on MHT. Of course she didn't, because she is a wonderful healer who has never judged me for anything I've shared with her. She told me she had several clients who had found relief upon starting MHT.

I expected my brother and his wife – both physicians (my sister-in-law is a specialist in obstetrics and gynaecology) – to judge me for starting MHT and regale me with warnings and alarms. Of course they didn't. They told me they were glad I had found relief.

I expected my parents, retired physicians, to judge me for starting MHT and warn me off it. Of course they didn't. They asked me if it was helping me and said they were glad when I said it was.

I understood that the only person judging me for starting MHT was me. Seven weeks into MHT, I am still arguing with myself about MHT.

I had not taken the time to separate strength and ageing from suffering.

It feels indulgent to talk about suffering as Israel continues its genocide in Gaza; as the suffering in Sudan and Congo and too many other places reminds us again and again of the toll on those who walk through the world and are not white, able-bodied and affluent cis-het men.

In so many of the life narratives given or allowed to cisgender women, suffering equates strength. Those social scripts signal to us that we've 'failed at womanhood' if we don't plough through suffering.

What is a 'strong' woman? How does a 'strong' woman navigate the menopause transition? How does a feminist navigate menopause? What is a feminist menopause?

I'm working on it!

Strength training, which I started in October 2022, a month before I became postmenopausal, helped me separate 'strong woman' from suffering; to point to the ever-increasing weights and say, 'There! I am strong,' thus liberating myself from having to prove anything . . . to who? To me? I am the strongest, physically, I've ever been. I can deadlift more than my body weight and I can squat close to my body weight.

Nonetheless, as exhilarating as it is to stand before a barbell that weighs more than you do and, with proper breathing and form, lift it, again and again, I could not deadlift my way to writing. I could not squat the words out of me.

Who was I when I was not a writer?

Perhaps that's exactly what menopause was designed to do all along – to force you to confront what you thought was the very essence of you, what made you you, and to let it go. Because even if you don't let it go – can't, won't, don't want to – it will let you go, set you adrift, make you pause: pause to wander – in the ellipses that separate who you thought you were and the you that is yet to come; pause to wonder – who the fuck am I now?

Menopause. Monapause.

Because when you wander and wonder, you will meet previous iterations of you, and they will excitedly ask, 'What have we become? Show us!' Tell them who they led you to become, the way stars once led explorers, thank them for bringing you this far, for forming the constellation of you, and let them go.

And grieve.

It is no small thing to let go of your night sky. Astronomers have invented a new term to describe the pain associated with humanity's loss of a dark sky, stars and all, because of light pollution: 'noctalgia', meaning 'night grief'.[7]

We need a word (perhaps, but not always, one that ends in -algia, the Greek word for pain) for the grief of losing our past selves. We need a ritual that can serve as a baton connecting the ellipses between what we were and what we are becoming. My word is Monapause (I could not resist) and my ritual is tattooing (of course – have you seen me?).

One day in October last year, almost a year into my postmenopause, I stood in the tattoo space of the artist Mugen (@mugen_tattoo) as they performed a ritual smudging. As they surrounded me with the smoke of the herbs they were using for the smudging, I thanked the Monas who had brought me thus far. I told them I loved them for all they had done, and let them go. I accepted the baton they handed me across the ellipses of me and prepared for the next part of our relay.

And then Mugen tattooed two Ancient Egyptian wedjat eye amulets into my upper back. The wedjat eye 'embodies healing power and symbolises rebirth. An amulet in this shape was thought to protect its wearer and to transfer the power of regeneration onto him or her.'[8]

Under the eye on the right is a lion, symbolising Sekhmet, the lion-headed goddess of retribution and sex, who is tattooed into my right inner forearm. Under the eye on the left is a cow, for Hathor, the goddess of love, beauty, music and pleasure. She is, at times, considered the more mature aspect of Sekhmet.

They are looking at each other on my upper back: Sekhmet handing me over to Hathor, bridging the ellipses of Mona.

By the time I was at my gynaecologist's clinic to start MHT, I was ready.

This essay took longer to write than usual. But I've learned to let go of 'usual', letting it fall in between the ellipses of me. And that has taught me a new way to be – to take my time. This essay is halting and faltering and raw – like the birds I heard during one of my walks in the park, whose chirping tentatively asked, 'Is this spring?' All I could hear was, 'Listen, I love you, spring is coming.' (A riff on a line from Kim Addonizio's poem

'To the Woman Crying Uncontrollably in the Next Stall': 'listen I love you joy is coming'.⁹)

I did not start MHT so that I could 'go back to normal' or 'go back to myself'. The self is not a static point in time, but rather an evolution of selves, an evolution of Monas that brought me to where I am now and said, 'Go! Live! Live well.' And I thank them for that evolution. Thank you. I've got it. I'll take it from here.

That's what I believe menopause hormone therapy has allowed to happen – for me to continue from the point where they led me to. So that I can live well in the time ahead of me. Not to go back to anything, but to move forward towards what is to come. When I started MHT, I understood how sensitive I was to hormonal shifts in my body and it brought into sharp relief, through the relief it brought me, just how shit I felt, and for how long I've felt shit.

Is this the second spring, as traditional Chinese medicine calls the menopause transition?

Listen, I love you, spring is coming.

Mona Eltahawy
March 2024

Notes

The Menopause: When We Are Free

1. Dr Jen Gunter, *The Menopause Manifesto: Own Your Health with Facts and Feminism*, New York: Citadel Press/Kensington Publishing Corp., 2021.
2. Kristen Hawkes, 'The grandmother effect', *Nature* 428, pp. 128–9 (2004), doi.org/10.1038/428128a
3. Tabitha M. Powledge, 'The Origin of Menopause: Why Do Women Outlive Fertility?', *Scientific American*, 3 April 2008, www.scientificamerican.com/article/the-origin-of-menopause/
4. David P. Barash, 'The Evolutionary Mystery of Menopause', *Nautilus*, 9 August 2022, nautil.us/the-evolutionary-mystery-of-menopause-238527/
5. Gunter, *The Menopause Manifesto*, Introduction.
6. Vanita Singh and M. Sivakami, 'Normality, Freedom, and Distress: Listening to the Menopausal Experiences of Indian Women of Haryana', in Chris Bobel, Inga T. Winkler, Breanne Fahs, et al. (eds.), *The Palgrave Handbook of Critical Menstruation Studies*, Singapore: Palgrave Macmillan, 2020. Chapter 70. Available from: www.ncbi.nlm.nih.gov/books/NBK565663/ doi: 10.1007/978-981-15-0614-7_70
7. Srilatha Batliwala, *All About Power: Understanding Social Power & Power Structures*, 10 May 2019, grassrootsjusticenetwork.org/resources/all-about-power-understanding-social-power-power-structures/
8. 'Average life expectancy at birth in Africa for those born in 2023, by gender and region', Statista, www.statista.com/statistics/274511/life-expectancy-in-africa/

9 'Average life expectancy at birth in Asia for those born in 2023, by gender and region', Statista, www.statista.com/statistics/274516/life-expectancy-in-asia/
10 World Health Organization, 'Menopause: Key Facts', 17 October 2022, www.who.int/news-room/fact-sheets/detail/menopause
11 World Economic Forum, 'This is how women's rights have progressed', 6 March 2020, www.weforum.org/agenda/2020/03/international-womens-day-equality-rights/
12 HelpAge International, 'Consortium Press Statement on Lynching of Elderly Women in Gusiiland', www.helpage.org/silo/files/consortium-press-statement-on-lynching.pdf
13 HelpAge International, 'Violence against older women: tackling witchcraft accusations in Tanzania', social.un.org/ageing-working-group/documents/HelpAge%20briefing%20violence%20against%20older%20women%20Aug%2011.pdf
14 Katy Migiro, 'Despite murderous attacks, Tanzania's "witches" fight for land', Reuters, 21 March 2017, www.reuters.com/article/us-tanzania-women-landrights-idUSKBN16S2HU

Bits of Flesh: For Anarcha – From Enslavement to Menopause

1 Omisade Burney-Scott, *Messages from the Menopausal Multiverse*, Black Girl's Guide to Surviving Menopause, Durham, NC, 2020.

The Curse of Puberty

1 Christy Harrison, *Anti-Diet: Reclaim Your Time, Money, Well-Being and Happiness Through Intuitive Eating*, Great Britain, Yellow Kite, 2019.
2 J. J. Brumberg, *The Body Project: An intimate history of American girls*, New York: Random House, 1997.
3 A. M. Gustafson-Larson and R. D. Terry, 'Weight-related behaviors and concerns of fourth-grade children', *J Am Diet Assoc.*, July 1992, 92 (7), pp. 818–22, PMID: 1624650.

4 C. A. Houston et al., 'Eating disorders among dietetics students: an educator's dilemma', *J Am Diet Assoc.*, April 2008, 108 (4), pp. 722–4. doi: 10.1016/j.jada.2008.01.048. PMID: 18446990.

I Don't Like Being Late: An Experience of Perimenopause From Turkey

1 Nilgün Marmara, 'Beden', *Daktiloya Çekiliş Şiirler*, Everest Yayınları, 2006 (quoted fragment translated by Canan Marasligil).
2 Aslı Alpar (ed.), *Jinekolog Muhabbetleri (Conversations at the Gynaecologist)*, Kaos GL Derneği, 2020, kaosgldernegi.org/images/library/2020jinekolog-muhabbetleri-son.pdf
3 'Erken menopozu deneyimleyenler anlatıyor: Bilgi verilmiyor, öneriler gebe kalmaya teşvikle sınırlı!' ('Those who have experienced early menopause talk: No information, only recommendations to conceive!'), kaosgl.org/gokkusagi-forumu-kose-yazisi/erken-menopozu-deneyimleyenler-anlatiyor-bilgi-verilmiyor-oneriler-gebe-kalmaya-tesvikle-sinirli
4 'Erkek şiddetinin 2022 videosu ve infografiği' ('2022 Video and Infographics of Male Violence'), Bianet, bianet.org/bianet/toplumsal-cinsiyet/273987-erkek-siddetinin-2022-videosu-ve-infografigi
5 ILGA-Europe Annual Review 2023, www.ilga-europe.org/report/annual-review-2023/
6 Global Gender Gap Report 2023, World Economic Forum, www3.weforum.org/docs/WEF_GGGR_2023.pdf
7 Türkiye'de kadın sağlığı | Yasal kürtaj hakkında engellemeler: 'Benim bedenim, kimin kararı?' (Women's Health in Turkey | Barriers to legal abortion: 'My body, whose choice?', www.youtube.com/watch?v=fuB_yjlbc-A

Sex and the Menopausal Vagina in the Suburbs

1 Shema Tariq et al., *PRIME (Positive Transitions Through the Menopause) Study: a protocol for a mixed-methods study investigating the impact of the menopause on the health and well-being of women living*

with HIV in England, BMY Open, bmjopen.bmj.com/content/9/6/e025497
2 'Is childbirth more dangerous for Black women in the UK?', Open Access Government, 23 May 2022, www.openaccessgovernment.org/childbirth-black-women-uk/117437/
3 Jacob Smith, 'New analysis reveals Black women in England more likely to be diagnosed with late-stage cancer', Cancer Research UK, 27 January 2023, news.cancerresearchuk.org/2023/01/27/new-analysis-reveals-black-women-in-england-more-likely-to-be-diagnosed-with-late-stage-cancer/

Feeling OldCute. Might Delete Later

1 Susan Dominus, 'Women Have Been Misled About Menopause', *New York Times*, 1 February 2023, www.nytimes.com/2023/02/01/magazine/menopause-hot-flashes-hormone-therapy.html

A Field Guide to Menopause

1 Monica Ploetzke, 'Fibroids: Greater in African-American Women than White. Why?', McLeod Health, www.mcleodhealth.org/blog/fibroids-greater-in-african-american-women-than-white-but-why/#

Free Fall

1 Syd Yang, 'Blood Memory', 2017.

Afterword

1 Mona Eltahawy, 'Moisturize Your Vagina', FEMINIST GIANT, 17 October 2021, www.feministgiant.com/p/moisturize-your-vagina?r=5ole&utm_campaign=post&utm_medium=web

2 Mona Eltahawy, 'Menopause is Shit. Menopause is Amazing', FEMINIST GIANT, 19 September 2022, www.feministgiant.com/p/essay-menopause-is-shit-menopause?r=5ole&utm_campaign=post&utm_medium=web

3 Alisha Haridasani Gupta, 'Study Shows the Staggering Cost of Menopause for Women in the Work Force', *New York Times*, 8 May 2023, www.nytimes.com/2023/04/28/well/live/menopause-symptoms-work-women.html

4 Mona Eltahawy, 'The Power and Glory of Menopause', FEMINIST GIANT, 25 October 2022, www.feministgiant.com/p/essay-the-power-and-glory-of-menopause?r=5ole&utm_campaign=post&utm_medium=web

5 Aliyah Frumin, 'The very real impact menopause has on women's advancement in the workplace', MSNBC, 26 September 2023, www.msnbc.com/know-your-value/health-mindset/very-real-impact-menopause-has-women-s-advancement-workplace-n1307216

6 Sharon Malone and Jennifer Weiss-Wolf, 'America lost its way on menopause research. It's time to get back on track', *Washington Post*, 28 April 2022, www.washingtonpost.com/opinions/2022/04/28/menopause-hormone-therapy-nih-went-wrong/

7 Paul Sutter, 'The loss of dark skies is so painful, astronomers coined a new term for it', Space.com, 8 September 2023, www.space.com/light-pollution-loss-dark-skies-noctalgia

8 Wedjat Eye Amulet, The Met, www.metmuseum.org/art/collection/search/550997

9 Kim Addonizio, 'To the Woman Crying Uncontrollably in the Next Stall', poetrysociety.org/poems/to-the-woman-crying-uncontrollably-in-the-next-stall

Acknowledgements

I am so proud of this anthology and my biggest thanks go to the magnificent contributors who so generously shared their menopause transitions and to Sheyam Ghieth whose glorious art brings power and beauty to this collection.

Thank you the Unbound team for your love and support that made this anthology possible: John Mitchinson, Katy Guest, Aliya Gulamani and Flo Garnett.

Love for my beloved Robert E. Rutledge for walking with me on my menopause adventure.

And to everyone who pledged: immense gratitude and appreciation for your support. Special thanks to Ruth Ann Harnisch and Ruth Ann Subach: the most generous patrons.

Unbound is the world's first crowdfunding publisher, established in 2011.

We believe that wonderful things can happen when you clear a path for people who share a passion. That's why we've built a platform that brings together readers and authors to crowdfund books they believe in – and give fresh ideas that don't fit the traditional mould the chance they deserve.

This book is in your hands because readers made it possible. Everyone who pledged their support is listed below. Join them by visiting unbound.com and supporting a book today.

Chance A-R
Pam Abbott
Kirzten Achtelik
Martha
   Adam-Bushell
Audrey Adams
Sheila Addison
Amy Agigian
AJ
Chioma
   Akamnonu
Wilhelmena and
   Rhona Allin
Courtney Allison

Christine Altman
Jean Amaral
Samantha Amenn
Lynn Anair
Elizabeth Anders
Fiona Anderson
Dee Andrews
Mary Antonia
   Andronis
Jenna Appleton
Nikki Armstead
Philip Arny
Nidhi Arora
Mary Arras

Audra Aulabaugh
Erin B.
Sam Baker
Nancy Barich
Suswati Basu
Caroline Bate
Kate Baty
Val
   Bayliss-Brideaux
Kristin Beck
Teri Bedard
Emira Benfaiza
Fiona Berry
Suzanne Bertolett

SUPPORTERS

Sasha Bhat
Carey Bidtnes
Marja Bijl
Kate Birch
Kate Fucking
 Bisby
Iben Bjørnsson
Carolyn Black
Brandi Blackburn
Robin Blackburn
Anna Blake
Jean Blanks
Eve Blatt
Claire Bloom
Linda Blount
Abbie Blumberg
Whitney Erin
 Boesel
Cate Teuten Bohn
Aly Bonomini &
 Julia Willis
Enfys Book
Harriet Booth
Holly Bornemeier
Sari Botton
Eileen M
 Bradshaw
Anna Brent
Patricia Bresnan
Cara Brockbank
Sarah Brooks
Tina Brooks
Cheryl Brown
Ali Brumfitt
Erika Villarreal
 Bunce
Lynne Bundesen
Emily Burn
Alexandra Bury
Megan Butler
Cindy Butts
Conor Byrne
Elizabeth Cafferty
Elen Caldecott
Jay Calderisi
Kellie Carbone
Allyssa Carlton
Elinor Carmi
Beverley
 Carrington
Leslie Tark Carver
Linda Aklundh
 Cassar
Jemma Cassidy &
 Team 1821
Joanne Cavan
Karin Celestine
Edward Chapman
Katie N
 Chaumont
Lisa Chensvold
Iqra Choudhry
Eileen Chow
Theresa Christiani
Marie-Gwénaëlle
 Chuit
Jenna Clark
Jennifer Clark
L Clark
Susan B. Clark
Gaynor Clarkson
Sarah Clarry
James
 Clive-Matthews
Carole Clohesy
Eavan Coakley
Chey and Stephen
 Cobb
Beth Cockrell
Kate Codrington
Risa Cohen
Kirsten Cole
Maggie Cole
Rachel Collins,
 Emma Somers
Mary Conger
Bríd Conneely
Lisa Connell
Marcia Connolly
Nick Cooper
Sara Cooper
Shawna Coppola
Mary Cosgrove

SUPPORTERS | 247

Emma Crawford
Juanita Crider
Cat Crossley
Julia Croyden
Kat Culyer
MK Czerwiec
Faten Dabis
Jennie Dailey-O'Cain
Angela Daly
C Davies
Julia Davis
Kat Day
Susie Day
Diana DeFrancesco
Gina DeMatteis
Grant Denkinson
Katy Derbyshire
Ellen Diamond
Yasmine Nasser Diaz, Julia Soto
Angela Dickson
Jennifer Dill
Baby Djojonegoro
Julianne Domeny
Sandie Donnelly
Lesley Dougan
Leslie Doyle
Sara Drake
Angela Dullaghan
K&S Durocher
Genevieve Eastabrook
Andrea Eastman
Antonia Echefu
Carrie Anne Eckmire
Erika Edqvist
Claire Edwards
Rachel Edwards
Sebastiaan Eldritch-Böersen
Em Eley
Sophie Ellgaard
Natalie Holme Elsberg
Brooke Emmel
Lacey England
Christopher Ervin
Gabriella Espinosa
A'Maya Ettien
Bernadine Evaristo
Shahed Ezaydi
Khadijah Fancy
Nadine Faraj
Angela Faustina
Leta Hong Fincher
Arlene Finnigan
Donna Fisher
Diana M. Fletcher
Bryce Fornes-Bates
Amy Fort
Clare Fowler
Melissa Fowler
Trevanne Foxton
Kim Faircloth Fraser
Piera Freccero
Gretchen Frey
from menarche to menopause\:
Majda Gama
Serena Garcia
Kyla Gardiner
Amy Garman
Diakhoumba Gassama
Caroline Gausden
Lisa Gemino
Claire Genevieve
Ali George
Louise Gibbard
Bruno Girin
Jacob Gloor
Liz Gloyn
Trudi Goels
Veta Goler
Gaije Gordon
Reiko Graham
TR Grand

Catherine Gregory
Emily Gresley
Katy Guest
Julie Guihen
Nicola Haggett
Kate Halabura
Fiona Hale
Emily Hall
Karen Hall
Verity Halliday
Mina Hamedi
Leah Hamilton
Elizabeth
    Hamilton-Pearce
Carole Landrith
Hanna
Dr. Megan Sluga
    Harbin
Donna
    Hardcastle
Kate Hardie
Ruth Harley
Shae Harmon
Ruth Ann
    Harnisch
Leah Harris
Sophie Harris
Jason Harrison
Arianne
    Hartsell-Gundy
Lisa Hauk-Meeker

Julia Haverstock
CS Hawk
Maria Hawkins
Jessica Hayes
Katie Hays
Katherine Heck
Lisa Heeps
Nanna
    Heidenreich
Sarah Helps
Christine Henry
Tracy Heuring
Em Hill
Jennifer Hill
Katja Hiltunen
Jane Hobson
Alberta Hodgson
Stephanie Fucking
    Hodgson
Matthew Hodson
Susanne Hofu
Lucy Holmes
Nicola Holt
Kerenza Hood
Camille Hook &
    Margaret Riedel
Diane Horvath
Beth Howe
Becky Hughes
Ken Hughes
Emma Humphries

Caroline Hunt
Zara Hurst
Jojo Huxster
Karrie Hyatt
Sladjana Ivanis
Jasmine J
Penny Jackson
Dyan Jayjack
Jedidja
Deborah Jermyn
Andrea Johnson
Stephanie A.
    Johnson
AJ Johnstone
Jory Jolivet
Mary
    Jordan-Smith
Dolly Joseph
Shona Kambarami
Bakita Kasadha
Jessica Lemieux
    Kaufmann
Suzanne Kavanagh
Lisa Keating
Heather Kelley
Cheryl Kellond
Kathleen Kelly
Ashley Kelmore
Suri Kempe
Sarah Kendzior
M Kent

SUPPORTERS | 249

Mary Keogh
Jasper Kettner
Ameel Khan
Karen Kinbar
Mandy Kirby
Sarah Klapperich
Katrin Klinger
Ashley Knight
Sarah Knowles
Melanie Koserowski
Jenny Krikava
Mark Kulkens
Nicola Kumar
Christine Kunkel
Rebecca L
Larisa LaBrant
Melissa LaFlamme
Maureen Lakes
Cheryl Ann Lambert
Amy Lamé
LaToya Larkin
Elana Leanna
Anna Lebacq
Fiona Lensvelt
Ellen Leonard
Shoshana Lev
Micky LeVoguer
Cecilia Córdova Liendo
Liza Lim
Michelle Lincoln
Corey Jo Lloyd
Camille Lofters
L. López
Gemma Loughran
Leila Luheshi
Aleksi Lukander
Leah Lundell
Jen Lunn
Eugene Lynch
Helen Lynch
Kate Macdonald
Mariam Magsi
Elaine Mai
Michelle Maitland
Kristen Majury
Catt** Makin
Mina and Sana Malik
Annetta Mallon
April Mallory
Melissa Mandell
Vesna Manojlovic
Elizabeth Marcon
Lara Marcon
Catherine Margaronis
Marilyn Dawn Marinopoulos
Jennifer Marsellis
Kate Marsh
Michelle Marshall
Nina Martinez
Linda Mason
Ruth Norman Mason
Stephanie Mason
Rose Matthews
Paula Maylahn
Holly McAdams
Rachel McArdle
Conor McBride
Meredith McCanse
Elizabeth McCarthy
Lawrence McCrossan
Laura Walker McDonald
Laura McGrath
Abby McGrory
Susan McIvor
Megan McKenzie
Mary-Anne McTrowe
Shannon Mechutan
Sonia Mehta
Lynne Mendoza
Julie Meredith

Lauren Fogel Mersy
Christina Meyer
Taraya Middleton
Leigh Ann Mike
Faith Miller
Rachel Miller
Tiffany Miller
Vickie Miller
Sasi Milmo
Ruth Milne
Nazia Mirza
Sairah Mirza
Amy Mitchell
Natasha Mitchell
John Mitchinson
Johanna Mizgala
Dee Montague
Max Mora
Eve Moran
Jenny Moran
Gabrielle Morgan
Jackie Morgan
Elaine Morin
Cari Morningstar
Sue Morón-García
Sarah Morton
Hiba Moustafa
Una Mullally
Xanthe Muller
Kat Munn
Luna Muñoz
Claire Murphy
Oonagh Murphy
Christopher Murray
Helga Murray
Rose Murray
Mary Nally
Carlo Navato
Martina Navratilova
Silvia Barbina Neisner
Lucy Neville
Njoki Ngumi
Stacey Nievweija
Alex Nightingale
Elina Nikulainen
Fiona Northing
Ally Nuttall
Nneka Nwokolo
Erin O'Connor
Lisa O'Connor
Sara O'Connor
Karen O'Sullivan
Nuala O'Sullivan
Juliet O'Brien
Osai Justina Ojigho
Charlie Oliver
Tru Olson
Maria Padget
Maja Pakulnis
Katy Palmer
Tamara Parker
Julie Parr
Larissa Parson
Julie Parsons
Jaqi Pascoe
Francesca Pashby
Chantal Patton
Melanie Peake
Lauren Pearce
Lydia Pearce
Eleanor Pender
Kate Permut
Charity A. Petrov
Debbie Phillips
Scout Phillips
Caroline Platt
Erika Polson
Alexandra Pope
Julieanne Porter
Reka Prasad
Susan Price
Tara Pritchard
Sarah Profit
Karen Pudner
Pun'kin
Emma Quigley
Valerie Quinn
M Rachlin

SUPPORTERS | 251

Heather Rai
Anna Rajendran
Amanda Ramsay
Krista Ranacher
Jillian Fucking
  Ratt
Meg Ray
Paula Read
S Reeson
Amber Regis
Kirsten Reynolds
Sarnata Reynolds
Anca Rightmire
Kerry Rini
Courtney
  Riseborough
Pamela Ritchie
Melissa RM
Beth Roberts
Charlotte
  Robertson
J Robinson
Rochelle Rochelle
Katie Roden
Louise Rolfe
Skylar Liberty Rose
Aron Lee
  Rosenberg
Beck Rosoman
Esther Roth
Marissa Rothkopf
Elsa Charlotte
  Rowe
Mills Rowe
Lucy
  Rowles-Springer
Adrienne Ruhnow
Lisa Rull
Caitlin Russell
Amanda Rutter
Gill Ryan
Helen Ryan
Deirdre
  Ryan-Knight
Nadi S
C N Sainsbury
Dorothea Salo
Marta Sampedro
Caroline
  Sanderson
Suzanne Sannwald
Davey Sawatzky
Shoshanna
  Sayeed-Smith
Ann Scanlan
Julie Scelfo
Sue Schmitz
Lisa Schneider
Fiona Scott
Kirsty Scott
Ashley E.
  Sepulveda
Marian Sexton
Maaza Seyoum
Rebecca Shadwick
Amy Shaiman
Lisa Shannon
Audrey Sharp
Frances Shaw
Therese Shechter
Maran Sheils
Dr. Sarah Shih
Kim Shoemaker
Kathryn Shovlin
Annapoorna
  Shruthi
Kym Silvasy-Neale
N J Simmonds
Kimberly
  Simmons
John Sindelar
Donna Sink
Ruby Sinreich
Beverley Slade
Elizabeth Slagus
Glen Sluga
Immy Smith
Nicole Smith
Ailbhe Smyth
Sylvia Solanas
Rachel Sollid
Joey Soloway
Esther Sparrow

252 | SUPPORTERS

Babs Spicer
Natalie Springhart
Nina Springle
Wendy Staden
Jane Stallman
L Stallman
Angela Stapleford
Stay Kind Universe
Miranda Stearn
Karyn Steers
Karen Steuer
Lorraine Stevenson
Jessica Stewart
Kate Stewart
Anita Stocker
Emma Jane Stone
Louie Stowell
Allison Strachan
Sophie Strachan
Jan Strain
Karla Strand
Cheryl Swift
Layla Tabatabaie, Esq.
Stephanie Tagtow
Dina A. Taha
Kathryn Tait
Mae Tang
Reem Taye
Megan Taylor
Susana Tempel
The Buddha Smiled
The Essence of Woerm Sin
Dana Theus
Didier Thevenard Thierna
Emma Thomas
Emma Daman Thomas
Isobel Thomas
Jane Melanie Thomas
Eaman Thompson
Kristen Thompson
Maria Markham Thompson
Fiona Thoms
Rachel Timbs
Ivana Tinkle
Mary Torres
Tishana Trainor
Ragini Tripathi
Lisa Tulfer
Duchess Umbrage
Sara Underwood
Deborah Vaile
Sarah Vaill
Valentina
Marieke Valstar
Abigail van Roode
Zach Van Stanley
Katina Velkou
Aparna Vengakkattu
Colleen Cary Verhey
Sarah Vidler
Babs Viejo
Athena Viscusi
Viola Strepsata Voltairine
Friederike von Lehe
Jennifer Wai
S Wake
Olivia Wakefield
Allison Walker
Charlotte Walker
Carla Ward
Gina Warren
Kellee Warren
Jennifer Webster
R Wechsler
Martha Weekes
Jacqueline Wernimont

Laura West
Carolee Gilligan Wheeler
Lucy Whitaker
Elizabeth White
Susan E. Wigget
Helen Wilde
Alison Williams
Laurynda Williams
Mark Williamson
Christina Willmore
A Winkworth
Elly Zoe Winner
Barrett Winston
Sydney Wise
Stacey Woods
Kristi Woolsey
Seren Worton
Hester P Wylde
Jennifer Wynne
Tahira Yaqoob
JA Young
Harriet Yudkin
Tarik Zahr
Hina Zaidi
Nilima Zaman
Jane Zibarras
Leni Zumas

A Note on the Type

Sabon is an old-style serif typeface designed in the mid-sixties by German-born typographer and designer Jan Tschichold (1902–1974). It is a classic typeface for body text, popular in book design.

Tschichold was commissioned by Walter Cunz at Stempel to design a new typeface, as requested by the German Master Printers Association, that could be printed identically on Linotype, Monotype or letterpress machines. The intention being to simplify the process of planning lines and pagination when printing a book.

The design of the roman is based on the classical types of Claude Garamond.